AI for Animals
Revolutionizing Veterinary Care

By
Amelia Hawkins

AI for Animals

Revolutionizing Veterinary Care

Table of Contents

Introduction

Picture a world where a veterinarian can diagnose a complex condition in a dog with just a smartphone or where surgical precision is enhanced by the guiding hand of a robotic assistant. Welcome to the transformative realm of artificial intelligence (AI) in veterinary medicine. While the notion of AI often conjures images of futuristic cityscapes and humanoid robots, its most profound and immediate impacts might be taking place on our farms, in our homes, and in veterinary clinics across the globe.

Veterinary medicine, an endeavor historically driven by keen observation and deep empathy, is on the cusp of a technological revolution. This field stands to gain immensely from AI's capabilities in data analysis, pattern recognition, and automation. Imagine the power of having access to a vast, interconnected web of knowledge that grows with each new case and is ever-ready to offer precise and objective support. This potentiality is what fuels the excitement surrounding AI's integration into animal care.

The impetus for adopting AI in veterinary medicine isn't merely rooted in the allure of technology, though. At its heart lies a more humane aspiration: to provide the best possible care for all creatures, great and small. As global awareness of animal welfare increases, so does our responsibility to employ every tool at our disposal, ensuring that treatments are not just adequate but exemplary.

For tech enthusiasts, veterinarians, and animal lovers alike, the convergence of AI and animal health care offers both a thrilling frontier and a pressing necessity. AI brings with it the promise of early disease detection, personalized treatment regimens, and unparalleled precision in surgeries. Yet, with these advancements come new questions about ethical considerations, the balance between technology and touch, and the best pathways to responsibly integrate AI into everyday practice.

Our journey through this exploration begins with understanding the essential components of AI and how they relate to the multifaceted field of veterinary medicine. From the basics of machine learning to implementing AI-driven diagnostic tools, the initial chapters lay a foundation for comprehending the deep-seated changes underway. We'll delve into AI's role in creating personalized treatment plans tailored to each animal's needs, ensuring not only efficiency but effectiveness in outcomes.

Surgery, too, is poised for transformation. With AI-assisted techniques and robotic precision, procedures are becoming safer and recovery times shorter. The ability to enhance surgical outcomes has the potential to mitigate pain, reduce complications, and ultimately save lives.

Beyond the clinical walls, AI is charting new courses in research and development. This burgeoning field accelerates drug discovery and revolutionizes clinical trials, bringing next-generation medications to animals faster than ever before. Furthermore, the reach of telemedicine is expanding, bringing expert veterinary care to remote areas through virtual consultations and remote diagnostics, powered by sophisticated AI algorithms.

Even in the wild, AI's influence is felt as it monitors wildlife populations and aids conservation efforts. These technologies give conservationists the tools to understand and protect delicate ecosystems in unprecedented ways. This global footprint of AI underscores its versatility and necessity in modern veterinary practices, reaching insights and solutions once thought unattainable.

While AI introduces a new era, it also demands thoughtful consideration of ethical practices and the impact on the veterinary profession. Questions about data privacy, informed consent, and the potential widening of existing gaps in veterinary access must be addressed to harness AI's benefits responsibly.

The integration of AI into veterinary education serves as a cornerstone for preparing future veterinarians, equipping them with the skills necessary to navigate and lead in this digital age. AI-enhanced learning tools are not just supporting the current curriculum but also reshaping the learning experience itself, allowing for more diverse, efficient knowledge acquisition.

The financial landscape of veterinary practices is also under transformation. While initial investments in AI technologies can be substantial, the long-term cost savings, efficiency gains, and improved patient outcomes present compelling reasons for adoption. AI's potential to attract investments and open up new funding avenues marks a progressive economic influence on the industry.

As we unravel AI's role across various chapters of this exploration, each segment offers a glimpse into specific applications and case studies, illustrating the successes and lessons learned from AI-enhanced veterinary care. Whether you're a practicing veterinarian contemplating AI adoption, an animal lover curious about the future of pet care, or a technologist eager to explore AI's potential, there's an undeniable momentum at the intersection of AI and animal health.

As we stand on the brink of this technological frontier, the symbiotic relationship between AI and veterinary medicine beckons us to rethink possibilities, innovate with responsibility, and ultimately strive for a world where every animal receives the highest level of care possible. Such is the promise—and the challenge—of AI in veterinary medicine, a field that is not just evolving but is poised to redefine what's possible for every animal in our care.

Chapter 1:
Understanding AI in Veterinary Medicine

Embarking on the journey of AI in veterinary medicine reveals a landscape rich with innovation and potential. As AI technologies seamlessly blend into veterinary practices, they bring transformative changes that redefine the realm of animal healthcare. From sophisticated algorithms that enhance decision-making to machine learning models that tirelessly analyze patterns, AI offers unprecedented opportunities for improved diagnostics and treatments across diverse species. These intelligent systems empower veterinarians to deliver precise care, enabling earlier disease detection and personalized treatment that considers each animal's unique needs. As we stand at the cusp of this technological revolution, the synergy between AI and veterinary medicine not only promises to elevate the quality of care but also inspires a future where the health and welfare of animals can be safeguarded with greater foresight and sensitivity. This chapter sets the stage for exploring how AI is revolutionizing every facet of veterinary science and crafting a brighter, more informed path for animal health.

The Basics of AI and Machine Learning

Artificial Intelligence (AI) and Machine Learning (ML) are at the heart of a technological revolution that is reshaping how we perceive and interact with the world. At its core, AI refers to computer systems that can perform tasks typically requiring human intelligence. These tasks include problem-solving, recognizing patterns, and understanding natural language. Machine Learning, a subset of AI, enables systems to learn from data, improving their performance over time without being explicitly programmed. This learning capability is particularly transformative in fields like veterinary medicine, where the ability to process and analyze vast amounts of animal health data quickly and accurately is crucial.

In veterinary medicine, AI is not just a buzzword—it's a catalyst for change. From diagnosing complex diseases to predicting health outcomes, AI-powered tools provide unprecedented insights into animal health. Machine Learning models, trained on datasets gathered from various species and conditions, help veterinarians make informed decisions. These tools can automate routine tasks, allowing veterinarians to focus more on personalized patient care.

Understanding the intricacies of AI begins with data. Data is the life force that fuels AI systems. In the veterinary context, data comes from diverse sources: medical records, imaging results, lab tests, and even behavioral studies. Effective AI models require large volumes of high-quality data for training. The richer and more comprehensive the data, the more accurate and reliable the AI models become. Once trained, these models can identify patterns, anomalies, and trends that might elude the human eye, leading to faster and more accurate diagnostics.

Machine Learning operates through algorithms, which are sets of instructions that tell a computer how to process the data it's given. There are several types of Machine Learning algorithms, each suitable for different kinds of problems. Some of the most common algorithms used in veterinary medicine include supervised, unsupervised, and reinforcement learning. Supervised learning models are typically used when there is a labeled dataset available, meaning the desired output is known. This is particularly useful in disease diagnosis where known conditions need identification. Unsupervised learning is applied to data without predefined labels, discovering underlying patterns or groupings. This can be instrumental in behavior analysis or identifying unknown health conditions.

Reinforcement learning, on the other hand, teaches an agent to take actions in an environment to maximize cumulative rewards. It is crucial in developing AI systems that require decision-making over time, such as optimizing treatment protocols based on gradual feedback about an animal's response.

One pivotal concept in AI is neural networks, inspired by the human brain's network of neurons. These networks consist of layers of interconnected nodes, or 'neurons,' which process data in complex ways. Deep learning, a subfield of machine learning, uses neural networks with many layers—hence 'deep.' This structure allows the processing of high-dimensional data like images and sequences, making it suitable for interpreting medical images such as X-rays and MRIs for anomalies that suggest illness.

As AI systems become more advanced, their ability to understand natural language is improving. Natural Language Processing (NLP) is the branch of AI that focuses on the interaction between computers and humans through language. For veterinary medicine, NLP applications can be revolutionary in facilitating communication between veterinarians, analyzing clinical notes, and even translating animal behavioral signals into actionable data.

However, the power of AI and ML in veterinary medicine is not merely technological; it's profoundly empathetic. By augmenting the capabilities of veterinarians, these technologies free professionals to devote more time and attention to patient care. AI can take over labor-intensive data analysis, allowing veterinarians to concentrate on nurturing the bond between humans and animals—a bond that lies at the core of veterinary medicine.

The integration of AI into veterinary medicine is just beginning. Researchers are continually developing more sophisticated algorithms, expanding the scope of what AI can achieve. But with great power comes great responsibility. The ethical considerations of deploying AI in sensitive fields like veterinary healthcare are critically important. Ensuring data privacy, addressing biases in AI models, and maintaining a human touch in animal care remain vital as we embrace these innovations.

Ultimately, the promise of AI in veterinary medicine is immense. It has the potential to revolutionize how we understand animal health, deliver care, and improve outcomes across species. But realizing this potential requires a marriage of technical proficiency and compassionate care—ensuring that technology empowers veterinarians without overshadowing the irreplaceable human-animal bond.

In conclusion, the basics of AI and Machine Learning lay the groundwork for transforming veterinary practices. As we advance, the convergence of AI innovation and veterinary expertise will sculpt a bright future for animal healthcare. Through AI, we not only enhance our ability to care for animals but also deepen our understanding of the natural world, stewarding a journey of growth, empathy, and discovery in veterinary science.

Integrating AI into Veterinary Practices

As we delve into the intersection of technology and veterinary medicine, it's clear that AI stands at the forefront of transformative change. The integration of AI into veterinary practices is not merely about adopting new tools; it's about reshaping the delivery of care in ways that were once the realm of science fiction. The true promise of AI lies in its ability to enhance the capabilities of veterinarians, enabling them to provide more accurate diagnoses, personalized treatment, and innovative care methodologies.

Veterinary practices, much like their human healthcare counterparts, are seeing an influx of data every day. From clinical records and imaging results to genetic and behavioral data, the sheer volume can be overwhelming. This is where AI shines. By employing advanced machine learning algorithms, AI systems can analyze vast datasets to uncover patterns and insights that might elude human practitioners. The result is a more informed and timely decision-making process, ultimately leading to improved patient outcomes.

In practice, integrating AI involves aligning with existing workflows rather than overhauling them. For example, AI-powered diagnostic tools can seamlessly blend with current imaging technologies, offering veterinarians enhanced interpretative capabilities. Imagine an AI system that reviews x-rays or ultrasounds, highlighting anomalies and providing differential diagnoses. Such tools act not as replacements but as colleagues that amplify a veterinarian's expertise and instinct.

Furthermore, AI-driven platforms can streamline administrative duties, allowing veterinarians more time to focus on patient care. Through natural language processing, AI systems can transcribe and organize notes, manage patient records, and even automate appointment scheduling. By reducing clerical workloads, veterinary staff can concentrate on what they do best—caring for animals.

Adopting AI in veterinary contexts also offers significant benefits in monitoring animal health. Wearable technologies equipped with AI capabilities can continuously track vital signs and behavioral patterns, alerting veterinarians at the first sign of deviation. For instance, if a pet's heart rate increases beyond typical levels, the system can prompt a notification, facilitating early intervention. This kind of proactive care could be pivotal in preventing minor issues from becoming serious health problems.

Despite the many advantages, the integration of AI is not without its challenges. Veterinarians must navigate a landscape that includes not only technological adaptation but ethical considerations as well. It is crucial to ensure that AI enhances the veterinarian-client-patient relationship, rather than diminishing the human touch. Transparency in AI recommendations and decisions is vital to maintain trust within the veterinary community and with pet owners.

Moreover, training and education are key components in successful AI integration. Veterinary professionals must be equipped with the understanding and skills to leverage AI technologies fully. This demands a paradigm shift in veterinary education, incorporating AI literacy as a core component of the curriculum. The goal is to produce practitioners who are comfortable and confident in utilizing AI as a standard part of their diagnostic and treatment toolkit.

The financial implications of AI adoption in veterinary practices cannot be ignored. Implementing AI systems requires investment in software and possibly new hardware. However, when viewed through the lens of long-term benefits, such as increased efficiency, improved accuracy in diagnostics, and enhanced patient care, the return on investment is compelling. Practices geared towards innovation are more likely to attract tech-savvy clients seeking cutting-edge care for their beloved pets.

Ultimately, integrating AI into veterinary practices signifies a shift towards more data-driven, efficient, and personalized care delivery systems. It's a journey towards a future where veterinarians are supported by AI, allowing them to dedicate more time and energy to patient care and less to routine tasks. As technology continues to evolve, so too will its applications in animal health, opening doors to possibilities we are only beginning to imagine.

Chapter 2:
AI in Diagnostics

In the rapidly evolving landscape of veterinary medicine, AI in diagnostics stands out as a transformative force, fundamentally reshaping how veterinarians approach the detection and understanding of animal health issues. By harnessing the power of advanced algorithms and machine learning, AI enhances the diagnostic process, allowing for the swift and accurate interpretation of complex data that was once the realm of experienced specialists. Automated imaging and analysis have become indispensable tools, helping to identify diseases early when interventions are most effective. This leap forward not only accelerates the speed of diagnosis but also increases its precision, reducing the emotional and financial burdens on pet owners and veterinary clinics alike. As AI continues to integrate into diagnostic protocols, it offers the promise of more personalized and timely treatment plans, ensuring that our animal companions receive the highest quality of care possible. Through this breathtaking progress in technology, we envision a future where the mysteries of animal health are more transparent, and our ability to protect and heal those we cherish is profoundly enhanced.

Automated Imaging and Analysis

Automated imaging and analysis are heralding a new era in veterinary diagnostics, offering a transformative approach to how we understand and treat animal health. By leveraging the unprecedented capabilities of artificial intelligence, veterinarians can now hone in on details that human eyes might miss, accurately diagnosing conditions earlier and with greater precision. These advancements are powered by sophisticated algorithms that analyze vast amounts of imaging data to identify patterns and anomalies otherwise imperceptible, changing the very landscape of animal diagnostics.

Historically, the interpretation of medical images—such as X-rays, ultrasounds, and MRIs—relied heavily on the expertise and experience of veterinary radiologists. While human expertise remains invaluable, AI systems can analyze imagery at a scale and speed that humans simply can't match. These AI-powered tools act as a second set of eyes, examining minute details, enhancing contrasts, and discerning subtle changes in tissue or bone structures that can signify early stages of disease.

One of the most striking examples of AI in imaging is the early detection of diseases. For conditions like osteoarthritis and certain types of cancer, earlier diagnosis can significantly improve treatment outcomes. AI systems can be programmed to recognize biomarkers and disease indicators earlier than traditional methods, allowing veterinarians to implement treatment plans that might preempt more severe manifestations of the ailment. As a result, animals benefit from timely interventions that enhance their quality of life, and possibly, longevity.

The integration of AI into veterinary imaging isn't just about diagnostics; it's also about democratization of expertise. Rural vets and clinics without access to specialized radiologists can benefit from AI diagnostic tools, providing them with insights and analyses that might otherwise be unattainable. This accessibility ensures that quality care becomes a standard rather than an exception, irrespective of geographic and resource-related constraints, ultimately bridging gaps in veterinary medicine.

AI technology also enhances the educational aspects of veterinary medicine. Machine learning models powered by vast datasets can offer real-time feedback and training, helping veterinary professionals develop sharper diagnostic skills. These systems can identify knowledge gaps and suggest resources to improve understanding, thereby strengthening the capabilities of the workforce. Educational institutions have started harnessing these technologies, integrating them into curricula to prepare the next generation of vets for a future where AI complements their clinical acumen.

Despite the remarkable strengths of AI, challenges remain in its deployment. Data privacy is of paramount concern. Ensuring that imaging data is stored and used ethically and securely is essential to foster trust among practitioners and pet owners alike. Moreover, AI algorithms are only as good as the data they are trained on, necessitating diligent curation and updating of datasets to prevent biases and inaccuracies in diagnosis.

The ethical use of AI in imaging also raises questions about the role of the veterinarian. While AI excels in pattern recognition and data processing, it does not replace the nuanced judgment and empathy that a veterinarian provides. The ideal scenario sees AI as a partner in diagnostics, not a replacement for the human touch that is so crucial in caregiving.

Automation in imaging also presents financial implications for veterinary practices. While the initial setup and integration of AI technology can be costly, the long-term benefits include increased efficiency, accuracy, and ultimately, a reduction in costs associated with misdiagnosis or delayed treatment. Furthermore, as AI technology becomes more widespread and its benefits more apparent, veterinary practices might see an increase in clientele seeking advanced diagnostic capabilities.

Regulation and standardization of AI tools will be key to ensuring consistency and reliability across the board. This will require collaboration between veterinary professionals, regulatory bodies, and tech developers to establish guidelines and standards that maximize the utility of AI while ensuring high safety and ethical benchmarks are met.

In conclusion, automated imaging and analysis pave the way for a more precise, accessible, and efficient approach to animal healthcare. By harnessing the power of artificial intelligence, the veterinary field can move towards a future where timely, accurate diagnostics are the norm, enhancing the care provided to animals around the globe. As AI continues to evolve, the possibilities for improving animal diagnostics and treatments seem boundless, and it invites a promising future for veterinary medicine.

Detecting Diseases Early

In the realm of veterinary diagnostics, the early detection of diseases plays a pivotal role in the health and longevity of animals. Confident strides have been made through the integration of artificial intelligence, providing a level of precision and speed that was previously unimaginable. The ability to detect diseases early not only saves countless animal lives but also alleviates emotional and financial strains on pet owners and veterinary professionals alike.

Artificial intelligence has transformed diagnostics by analyzing data with incredible speed and accuracy. Diseases that were once detectable only in advanced stages can now be caught in their infancy through AI-enhanced tools. This revolution is largely attributed to the capability of AI to process vast amounts of data—from genetic profiles to behavioral patterns—and identify anomalies that may indicate the onset of illness.

One significant advancement lies in AI's ability to learn and predict patterns from historical data. Machine learning algorithms are trained on extensive datasets containing information about various diseases and their early biomarkers. With every new data point, these algorithms become smarter, enhancing their predictive accuracy over time. Consequently, veterinarians can make informed decisions faster, leading to timely interventions that can prevent severe complications or fatalities.

The implications of early disease detection are substantial in veterinary medicine, where time is often of the essence. AI enables veterinarians to identify conditions like cancers, heart diseases, or infectious diseases before they become critical. This helps in crafting more effective treatment strategies and improves prognosis significantly. The earlier the intervention, the better the chances of recovery and reduced suffering for the animal involved.

Moreover, AI-driven platforms often come integrated with user-friendly interfaces, enabling veterinarians to deliver more timely and efficient care. These systems offer an enhanced level of interactivity, providing real-time data analysis and insights that were once confined to the realm of expert interpretation. With these insights at their fingertips, veterinarians can focus on developing action plans rather than spending valuable time on manual data sorting and examination.

AI doesn't just empower professionals but extends its reach to animal owners as well. With AI-based applications and devices available, pet owners can participate actively in monitoring their pet's health. Wearable devices and smart sensors can track vital signs and behaviors, providing early warnings about potential health issues. These insights empower owners to seek professional help before a condition worsens, further underscoring the critical nature of early detection.

Despite the immense benefits, there is often skepticism surrounding the application of AI in veterinary practice, particularly regarding its reliability. Addressing these concerns is essential to gaining the trust of both veterinarians and pet owners. AI systems must be rigorously validated against a variety of scenarios to ensure they perform reliably under different conditions. Continuous updates and learning enhance the robustness of these systems, minimizing errors and maximizing accuracy.

Deploying AI in the early detection of diseases also invites ethical considerations. The reliance on technology calls for a balance between innovative benefits and ethical responsibilities. It becomes imperative for practitioners not only to harness these tools but also to maintain a vigilant oversight that upholds the compassionate care inherent in veterinary practices.

Furthermore, the integration of AI in diagnostics requires a reconsideration of traditional veterinary training. As AI tools become more prevalent, veterinarians must be equipped with the skills to utilize these technologies effectively. This shift calls for curricula updates and continuous education programs to ensure that future vets are as proficient with AI tools as they are with a stethoscope.

Collaborative efforts between AI experts and veterinarians are crucial in designing systems that meet the unique requirements of the veterinary field. Such collaborations ensure that the development of AI tools aligns with practical needs and ethical considerations while maintaining user-friendliness that facilitates widespread adoption.

Reflecting on these transformations, one cannot ignore the inspiring potential AI holds in the realm of veterinary care. As we continue to innovate, the promise of a future where diseases are routinely detected and addressed in their earliest stages is no longer just a dream but a fast-approaching reality. Embracing these advancements responsibly and ethically will pave the way for healthier animals and more fulfilled human-animal relationships.

Chapter 3:
Personalized Treatment Plans

In the evolving landscape of veterinary medicine, personalized treatment plans powered by AI stand at the forefront of transforming animal healthcare. Imagine a world where each animal receives a therapy perfectly tailored to its genetic makeup, lifestyle, and ongoing health data. This isn't just a futuristic fantasy—it's the reality that artificial intelligence is crafting. By harnessing vast datasets and identifying patterns that even the most experienced veterinarian might miss, AI allows for treatments that are both specific and dynamic, adjusting to the animal's changing needs. This proactive approach doesn't just enhance the efficacy of treatments; it revolutionizes the entire caregiving process, offering hope and improved outcomes for pet owners and veterinary professionals alike. The implications are profound: AI doesn't merely react to symptoms but anticipates them, thereby fostering an era of preventive care that truly looks after animals' long-term well-being and health. As we delve deeper into these capabilities, it's clear that personalized treatment plans signal a remarkable shift toward more compassionate and precise veterinary care.

Tailoring Therapies with AI

In the realm of veterinary medicine, personalization is more than just a trend; it's become a necessity. Every animal patient presents uniquely, with their own genetic makeup, lifestyle, environment, and health challenges. Here, AI steps in with its unparalleled ability to analyze vast amounts of data, ushering in a new era of tailored therapies that adapt to the specific needs of each animal. AI has begun to revolutionize the way veterinarians approach treatment plans, seeing beyond the surface to understand deeper nuances that influence health outcomes.

AI's contribution to personalized treatment goes beyond mere adjustments. By integrating data from various sources—such as genetic profiles, past medical history, current health stats, and even behavioral patterns—AI systems can generate comprehensive insights that drive more informed decisions. This dynamic approach not only matches treatments to specific conditions but also aligns them with the individual characteristics of the patient. It's like having a highly knowledgeable assistant who combs through endless datasets, correlating factors that even the most astute human eye might overlook.

Consider the process of diagnosing and treating a condition as complex as equine colic. A traditional approach might rely heavily on veterinarians' expertise and observations, but with AI, predictive analytics can play a pivotal role. AI models, trained on extensive datasets of historical cases, provide probabilities of specific causes for the symptoms observed. This predictive power can dramatically shift how treatment is administered, ensuring swift and effective interventions that are tailored for the individual horse's history and risk factors. As time progresses, AI systems become even more refined, continuously learning from new data, hence adapting alongside the evolving nature of medicine itself.

One groundbreaking aspect of AI in personalized treatments is its role in pharmacogenomics—the study of how genes affect a person's response to drugs—which can also be applied to animals. AI-driven pharmacogenomic analyses enable veterinarians to predict how an animal might respond to specific medications based on genetic information. This ensures that the right drug is administered at the right dose, minimizing adverse reactions and optimizing therapeutic efficacy. Imagine a scenario where a dog with epilepsy receives a drug regimen optimized just for his genetic profile, leading to a significant reduction in seizure frequency and severity without the troublesome side effects typically seen with a one-size-fits-all treatment.

Furthermore, AI can harness the power of machine learning to continuously monitor the effectiveness of treatment plans. This isn't about just setting and forgetting. By dynamically analyzing ongoing data from health monitoring devices and regular check-ups, AI systems can detect any deviations or inefficiencies in the current treatment strategy. These intelligent systems can suggest modifications or enhancements to the regimen, ensuring that interventions remain relevant and effective over time. Such adaptability ensures that the therapeutic journey aligns perfectly with the animal's changing needs and environments.

Let's also touch on the role of AI in rehabilitation therapy. For instance, AI's integration with physiotherapy allows for customized recovery programs that consider an animal's progress in real-time. By analyzing movement patterns and recovery metrics, AI can help design tailored exercises that facilitate optimal healing. This feedback loop empowers veterinarians and animal physiotherapists to refine rehabilitation strategies to speed up recovery times and enhance overall outcomes. An injured racehorse, for instance, might benefit from a customized AI-driven rehabilitation program that considers its athletic needs and past performance data for a speedy and safe return to the track.

Of course, personalization via AI extends beyond physical health to encompass mental and emotional well-being. Integrating AI tools with behavioral data can illuminate links between an animal's health and its environment, allowing for the adjustment of treatment plans to promote not just physical recovery but emotional and psychological healing as well. For animals experiencing anxiety or stress-related conditions, AI systems can recommend environmental or dietary modifications that cater to the specific triggers and needs of the individual animal. This holistic approach has the potential to improve quality of life significantly.

Despite these exciting advancements, it's essential to acknowledge the complexities and challenges associated with implementing AI-driven personalized therapies. The transition from conventional methods to AI-enhanced approaches requires not just technical adaptability but also a paradigm shift in mindset among veterinary professionals. As AI tools become more prevalent, veterinarians must be prepared to interpret AI insights critically, blending them with traditional assessment skills to achieve optimal results. It's a delicate balance where technology must enhance, not replace, the invaluable intuition and experience of skilled practitioners.

Ethical considerations also come into play. As we leverage AI to refine treatment protocols, it's crucial to ensure that this technology remains a tool for enhancing the caregiver-animal relationship, not overshadowing it. Transparency in how AI models function and the data they utilize must be maintained, fostering trust between veterinarians, pet owners, and the AI systems themselves. Moreover, inclusivity in the datasets used by AI is critical, ensuring that the algorithms are as unbiased and applicable across diverse animal population groups as possible.

In conclusion, the personalization of treatment plans through AI is a thrilling frontier that is rapidly transforming veterinary medicine. While challenges exist, the benefits of AI-driven tailored therapies are profound. The blend of detailed data analysis, predictive modeling, and real-time monitoring capabilities that AI offers is refining our approach to animal care. With AI as a partner in the veterinary field, the potential to significantly improve health outcomes for animals is more attainable than ever. This journey towards personalization in animal treatment is just beginning, but its trajectory is undeniably promising and poised to elevate animal healthcare to extraordinary new heights.

Monitoring and Adjusting Treatment

In the dynamic landscape of veterinary medicine, it's imperative that treatments don't remain static. Each animal, much like a human patient, presents a unique case that can evolve over time. This is where the concept of monitoring and adjusting treatment becomes crucial within the framework of personalized treatment plans. As we leverage artificial intelligence (AI) in veterinary practices, the potential for finely tuned, responsive treatments is more attainable than ever before.

AI-driven systems excel at processing vast amounts of data, enabling veterinarians to keep a watchful eye on treatment efficacy and make real-time adjustments. Consider a scenario where a dog diagnosed with a chronic condition undergoes a tailored treatment regimen. AI algorithms continuously analyze the animal's response to medications and suggest dosage changes or alternative therapies based on real-time data such as activity levels, dietary intake, and even subtle physiological changes captured by wearable devices. This adaptability ensures that treatment remains optimal, addressing the animal's evolving needs and minimizing the risk of adverse effects.

The integration of AI into monitoring tools transforms data from simple observations to actionable insights. For instance, intelligent systems can alert veterinarians if a prescribed treatment for arthritis in horses is not producing the desired improvement in gait. Such systems use wearable sensors to track movement patterns and analyze these against expected outcomes, allowing for timely intervention. This proactive approach not only enhances the animal's quality of life but also empowers veterinarians to provide more efficient and effective care.

Moreover, AI facilitates personalized treatment plans by enabling precision medicine, which refers to tailoring medical treatment to the individual characteristics of each patient. In veterinary medicine, this means considering the specific breed, age, weight, and genetic background of the animal. AI can analyze historical data related to similar patients and predict which treatments will work best for the current patient, essentially learning from past experiences to improve future outcomes.

When monitoring treatment efficacy, AI systems are particularly valuable in identifying subtle changes that human observation might miss. Machine learning algorithms can pick up on patterns and anomalies in an animal's behavior or biometric data. These systems learn to differentiate between normal variations and those that may indicate a need for a change in therapy. The continuous loop of monitoring, feedback, and adjustment allows for a more nuanced understanding of animal health.

Implementing these AI systems requires collaboration and trust between veterinarians and technology. Veterinary practitioners must feel confident in the AI systems they use, understanding their capabilities and limitations. Training and education play a pivotal role in this process. By empowering veterinarians with the skills to interpret AI-generated data and insights, they can make more informed decisions that enhance their practice and animal health outcomes.

The shift towards AI-enhanced monitoring also heralds changes in how treatments are conceptualized. Traditional treatment plans often rely on set intervals for evaluation and adjustment. However, with AI, the possibility of continuous assessment becomes feasible. This ongoing monitoring represents a paradigm shift where treatments are no longer bound by time-capsulated windows but are instead fluid, adjusting as needed. Such flexibility can be particularly beneficial in managing chronic conditions where treatment responses can vary widely among individual animals.

While AI introduces remarkable advancements, it's important to maintain a balanced approach. The veterinarian's expertise, empathy, and intuition remain irreplaceable. AI serves as an augmentation of their skills, offering additional layers of data and insight. Ultimately, the best outcomes arise from the synergistic relationship between human judgment and machine intelligence.

Incorporating AI into monitoring and adjusting treatment also contributes to cost efficiency. By minimizing trial-and-error approaches and optimizing medication dosages or therapy strategies, veterinary practices can reduce unnecessary expenditures. Furthermore, effective monitoring can result in shorter recovery times, thereby improving overall treatment efficiency and reducing long-term costs for pet owners.

The ethical considerations of AI in monitoring must also be addressed. Respecting animal privacy, ensuring data security, and promoting transparency in AI algorithms are crucial components of ethical AI practice. Trust between pet owners, veterinarians, and AI technology hinges on these principles. Open communication and clear explanations of how AI contributes to monitoring and treatment adjustments deepen this trust.

Looking ahead, the impact of AI on monitoring and adjusting treatment will likely expand. As AI technologies continue to evolve, the potential for integrating more sophisticated systems into routine veterinary practice grows. This evolution promises an era of veterinary care where treatment plans are as responsive and individual as the creatures they are designed to heal.

In conclusion, the role of AI in monitoring and adjusting treatment has shifted veterinary medicine towards a more dynamic, data-driven practice. It enhances the ability to deliver personalized and effective care, providing veterinarians with powerful tools to respond to the ever-changing health needs of animals. As AI technology advances, the horizon broadens, offering new possibilities for precision, compassion, and efficacy in animal healthcare.

Chapter 4:
Enhancing Precision in Surgery

The fusion of artificial intelligence with surgical practices in veterinary medicine is reshaping outcomes, offering unprecedented precision and reliability. As AI-assisted surgical techniques advance, veterinarians can perform intricate procedures with heightened accuracy, minimizing risks and maximizing recovery rates. Robots equipped with AI are not just futuristic concepts but practical tools, making meticulous incisions and delivering consistent results that surpass human limitations. Imagine the synchronicity of a veterinarian and AI working in tandem, refining the art of surgery to an innovative science. It's a harmonious dance of technology and expertise, empowering animal healthcare professionals to achieve feats that were once considered beyond reach. By embracing these technological advancements, the veterinary field takes a leap toward more effective, compassionate care, ensuring that animals receive optimal treatment that's less invasive and more effective in promoting their well-being.

AI-Assisted Surgical Techniques

In the rapidly evolving domain of veterinary medicine, AI-assisted surgical techniques have emerged as a transformative force, redefining precision and efficacy in procedures once constrained by human limitations. Artificial intelligence is not merely a tool; it's become a partner in the surgical suite, offering capabilities that enhance, optimize, and revolutionize the way veterinarians approach surgery. In AI-assisted surgeries, precision isn't just improved—it's elevated to levels previously unattainable.

The concept of AI in the operating room presents an intriguing interplay between human expertise and machine intelligence. Imagine a scenario where a complex surgery requires minute precision within fragile anatomical structures or demands swift decision-making in unexpected complications. In such cases, AI systems can support veterinary surgeons by providing real-time data analysis and predictive insights that can inform every snip, stitch, and suture. These systems, trained on vast amounts of surgical data, can predict potential challenges and suggest optimal pathways for surgical interventions, leading to outcomes that are less invasive and more effective.

Machine learning algorithms have come to play a critical role in pre-surgical planning. Before a single incision is made, AI can assist in creating a three-dimensional model of the animal's anatomy, offering a comprehensive map of its unique physiology. This allows surgeons to plan with unprecedented accuracy, identifying the exact location of tumors or malformations. Not only does this reduce surgical time, but it also minimizes trauma by curtailing unnecessary dissection, which can reduce recovery times and lower the risk of complications.

Another cornerstone of AI-assisted surgical techniques is robotic-assisted surgery, which is increasingly becoming integral to modern veterinary operating rooms. These robotic systems, guided by AI, assist veterinarians with precision that's unparalleled by human hands. For example, in delicate operations involving the spine or brain, robotic arms can hold surgical instruments steady, reducing the tremor and fatigue that can accompany prolonged procedures. Additionally, such robotics are equipped with visual feedback systems that enhance the surgeon's ability to perform microsurgeries with a level of detail that magnifies the surgical field far beyond human capability.

One can't overlook the role of AI in enhancing surgical training. For veterinarians embarking on their careers, AI-driven simulators offer rich, immersive experiences that mimic real-life scenarios without risk to animal patients. These simulators can adapt to the user's skill level, presenting varied complications to build decision-making skills and confidence. By doing so, AI not only aids in refining the technical prowess of future surgeons but also imbues them with a more profound understanding of surgical strategy and patient care, ultimately raising the standard of veterinary surgeries across practices.

Intraoperative decision support systems powered by AI mark another leap forward. As surgeries unfold, these systems continuously analyze data from vital signs, procedural progress, and even surgical tool interactions. They alert surgeons to potential issues such as incipient bleeding or equipment malfunction while suggesting corrective measures drawn from a database of past successful surgeries. Such apps and systems ensure that every moment of a procedure is backed by data-driven support, improving the chances of a successful and smooth operation.

AI-assisted surgical techniques are also revolutionizing postoperative care. Through algorithms trained on extensive surgical recovery data, AI provides insights into optimal recovery pathways tailored to each patient. This enables a bespoke rehabilitation process, which can significantly enhance healing efficiency, ensuring that animals return to their everyday lives quicker and with minimized post-surgical pain or complication risks. Additionally, AI can monitor post-operative recovery through wearables or smart devices, tracking vital signs and alerting caregivers to any deviations that require attention.

Progress isn't without its challenges, though. The integration of these technologies calls for an ethical consideration of their roles and a discussion about the evolving relationship between human veterinary surgeons and AI. It's crucial that these technologies remain tools for enhancement, not replacement. Trust must be established, ensuring that AI acts as an aid that enhances human judgment and compassion. After all, the heart of veterinary care lies in the empathetic connection veterinarians share with their animal patients—a bond AI can support but never replicate.

As AI continues to grow in capability, what seems almost certain is a future where surgeries become even more precise and less invasive. It's a vision where each procedure is not only a technical achievement but also a compassionate commitment to elevating the standard of care. AI-assisted surgical techniques promise not only to enhance surgical precision but also to transform the landscape of veterinary healthcare, opening the door to endless possibilities for improved animal welfare and surgical success. The ongoing collaboration between AI and veterinary surgeons signals a remarkable era of advancement with benefits reaching far beyond the operating table.

Improving Outcomes with Robotics

In the evolution of modern veterinary medicine, the integration of robotics into surgical procedures stands as a pioneering achievement. Robotic systems have revolutionized the domain of surgery, offering unprecedented levels of precision, control, and outcome predictability that were previously unattainable through traditional methods. The fusion of AI with robotics harnesses the power of precision, ushering in a new era where even the most delicate operations can be performed with meticulous care.

Robotics in veterinary surgery leverages mechanical efficiency and AI to enhance surgical performance across a broad spectrum of procedures. Unlike human surgeons, robotic systems are unencumbered by fatigue and are designed to perform with unwavering steadiness. This technology supports veterinarians by escalating their capabilities, not replacing them. It empowers them to undertake intricate surgeries with refined accuracy, ultimately aiming to minimize risks and maximize the efficacy of therapeutic interventions.

Take, for instance, the robotic-assisted surgical systems that are currently in use. These systems incorporate robotic arms equipped with tools that are articulated precisely to the needs of the surgery. The development of haptic feedback systems has been particularly impactful. These mechanisms provide real-time sensory feedback to the surgeon, allowing them to "feel" the surgical environment indirectly. This creates a tactile bridge between the surgeon and the robotic apparatus, enhancing the surgeon's ability to navigate complex anatomical structures with a reassuring delicacy.

Additionally, robotics mitigate the inherent limitations of human dexterity. For surgeries that demand the utmost precision, such as neurological or ophthalmic procedures, even the slightest hand tremor can compromise outcomes. Robotic systems neutralize these issues by providing controlled, tremor-free motions. This precision transforms challenging surgeries into feasible endeavors, broadening the scope of what veterinary surgeons can confidently address.

The synergy between robotics and AI introduces another layer of sophistication. AI algorithms can assist by analyzing pre-surgical imaging data to map out optimal surgical pathways. By simulating various scenarios, AI can suggest approaches that minimize tissue damage and optimize healing. This data-driven guidance supports the surgeon's decisions, enhancing the comprehensive planning of complex procedures and fostering a proactive approach to surgical challenges.

Moreover, the capacity for robotics to undertake minimally invasive surgeries has considerably reduced recovery times and postoperative complications. Traditional surgeries often involve substantial incisions, which can lead to longer healing periods and increased discomfort for the animal. In contrast, robotic-assisted surgeries require smaller incisions, which diminishes the trauma to surrounding tissues and promotes faster recovery. This advancement is crucial not only for the animal's welfare but also for the economic considerations of pet owners and veterinary institutions.

In equipping veterinary professionals with these cutting-edge tools, the focus naturally swings towards improving the quality and range of care available. For instance, robotic systems have been effectively deployed in orthopedic surgeries, facilitating precise bone cutting and alignment processes. This precision plays a critical role in ensuring successful outcomes in cases such as fracture repair or joint replacement, where alignment accuracy is paramount.

It's also worth noting that as more veterinary practices adopt robotic systems, the overall costs can be offset by the efficiencies gained. Shorter surgeries with fewer complications and quicker recoveries foster operational efficiency. Over time, this technology can provide savings that can be redirected towards broader adoption and further technological improvements. This positive feedback loop benefits both practitioners and patients, making high-quality veterinary surgical care more accessible and abundant.

The advent of robotics in surgery also opens up possibilities for innovative research and development. By analyzing the data generated from robotic procedures, researchers can identify patterns and outcomes that lead to further refinements in techniques and technology. This iterative process paves the way for continuous enhancement in surgical methodologies, driven by real-world insights and results.

Let's not overlook the educational implications. Training veterinary professionals on these systems is an integral part of their integration into practice. Simulation and training programs are essential to ensure that surgeons are proficient with the technology and can fully exploit its potential. As veterinary students and seasoned professionals alike become conversant with these systems, the collective competence within the field grows, which in turn raises the standard of care available worldwide.

In conclusion, the infusion of robotics into veterinary surgery is not merely an enhancement of existing practices but a transformative leap forward. The precision and reliability offered by robotic systems directly translate to improved surgical outcomes and heightened patient safety. As veterinary medicine continues to evolve, embracing innovative technologies such as robotics will be paramount in pushing the boundaries of what can be achieved, ensuring that our animal companions receive the best possible care in their time of need. This synergy of technology and care is an inspiring testament to the boundless possibilities that lie at the intersection of robotics and veterinary science.

Chapter 5:
AI-Driven Research and Development

As we shift our focus from the surgical suite to the research lab, the pivotal role of AI in revolutionizing veterinary medicine becomes even more apparent. This chapter highlights how AI is catalyzing breakthroughs in drug discovery and transforming clinical trial processes. By leveraging machine learning algorithms, researchers can now expedite the identification of promising compounds, considerably reducing the time and cost associated with traditional approaches. In clinical trials, AI models are being used to simulate outcomes and optimize test parameters, ensuring that trials are both efficient and robust. These advancements not only accelerate the introduction of new treatments but also enhance their precision and efficacy. Through AI-driven research, we're unlocking new possibilities in animal healthcare, offering unprecedented hope for veterinarians and animal lovers alike, as we stand on the cusp of groundbreaking medical innovations that could redefine animal well-being.

Innovative Drug Discovery

The ongoing evolution of artificial intelligence (AI) has begun to revolutionize the landscape of drug discovery, bringing unprecedented changes to the veterinary world. Historically, the development of effective medications for animals was both a time-consuming and costly endeavor. Traditional methods required years of research and testing, with significant financial investment before a new drug ever reached the market. But with AI driving innovation, the processes of discovering, designing, and testing new pharmaceuticals are seeing dramatic improvements in efficiency and effectiveness.

AI's ability to analyze vast datasets quickly and accurately plays a pivotal role. By sifting through extensive libraries of chemical compounds and biological data at an extraordinary pace, AI can identify potential drug candidates with promising therapeutic benefits. This pattern recognition prowess allows researchers to explore complex biological pathways and predict how different compounds might interact with veterinary patients, pointing scientists toward the most promising options for further study. It's like having a seasoned detective crack convoluted cases in a fraction of the usual time, amplifying the potential for breakthroughs we once thought improbable.

The transformative impact of AI in this realm is not just theoretical. Recent developments have shown how AI can predict animal disease models and simulate various scenarios with remarkable accuracy. These simulations can indicate how a new drug may affect specific species or cater to certain conditions, reducing the reliance on trial-and-error methods that previously dominated the field. The insights generated through these AI algorithms significantly trim the huge burden of early-stage failures, saving both time and resources. Moreover, AI-assisted drug discovery has proven beneficial in the creation of specialized drugs for rare or difficult-to-treat conditions. By cultivating an environment where niche treatments can be developed more viably and rapidly, AI fosters more personalized care solutions for animals in need.

One area where AI particularly shines is in the identification of correct dosage forms and routes of administration tailored to the unique physiology of different animal species. Differences in metabolism, body size, and organ function can significantly influence how animals process drugs, and AI tools are adept at optimizing these factors. As a result, veterinarians can provide more precise treatments, improving outcomes and minimizing side effects. The ultimate goal is personalized medicine, where every treatment plan is not just specific to a species but individualized to each patient.

Moreover, AI has opened doors for the utilization of big data in tracking disease patterns and drug resistance, a critical factor in today's global health climate. With the capability to analyze and learn from vast amounts of historical and real-time data, AI systems can develop predictive models that foresee how diseases might evolve or spread. This foresight aids researchers in designing more agile and anticipatory pharmaceutical strategies, preemptively tackling potential crises before they escalate. The integration of AI into epidemiological studies offers powerful tools for understanding and combating zoonotic diseases, which often lie at the intersection of human and animal health.

The collaborative potential of AI can't be overstated, offering excellent opportunities for partnerships between tech developers, veterinarians, pharmacologists, and researchers. By sharing insights and data across disciplines, the collective knowledge base expands exponentially. This collaboration accelerates the pace of discovery and innovation, while also fostering a supportive ecosystem where various stakeholders work toward common goals. As such, the entire drug discovery process becomes more efficient, with a creative and cooperative spirit driving the veterinary industry forward into uncharted territories.

Despite these promising advances, challenges remain. The ethical considerations of AI's role in drug discovery persist, particularly concerning data privacy and the accuracy of predictive models. It's vital to ensure that AI-driven research aligns with regulatory standards and ethical frameworks, maintaining transparency and reliability in all operations. Vetting and validating AI-generated results through rigorous scientific methods remain essential to confirm their efficacy and safety before being integrated into practice.

Another issue confronting the AI-driven drug discovery process is ensuring equitable access to these innovations. Effective dissemination of AI-developed drugs, especially in under-resourced areas, needs attention so that the animals globally can benefit from advances in veterinary pharmaceuticals. This balance between innovation and accessibility is crucial for ensuring that the full potential of AI is realized and that its benefits are felt across diverse animal populations.

The journey of AI in innovative drug discovery is only beginning, and yet its impact on the field is already palpable. By driving more efficient research and supporting the development of effective, targeted treatments, AI is poised to significantly advance veterinary medicine. As these tools and methods continue to evolve, so too does the possibility of a future where animal healthcare is not only reactive but profoundly proactive and personalized. The promise of this technology offers hope for healthier, happier animals paired with improved outcomes, sparking inspiration in what lies ahead in the world of veterinary pharmaceuticals.

Revolutionizing Clinical Trials

In the realm of veterinary medicine, clinical trials have traditionally been a lengthy and complex process. However, the integration of artificial intelligence (AI) into these trials is transforming the landscape dramatically. AI is streamlining every stage, from recruitment to data analysis, and is rapidly becoming indispensable. By employing machine learning algorithms and advanced data analytics, AI brings a new level of precision and efficiency to clinical trials typically reserved for human healthcare.

One of the most significant impacts of AI in clinical trials is its ability to enhance participant selection. Machine learning algorithms can analyze vast datasets to identify the most suitable candidates for trials based on a myriad of factors. This isn't just about choosing animals with the right medical conditions—it's also about considering genetic markers, historical health data, and even behavioral traits. By ensuring a match between participants and trials, AI minimizes variability and increases the likelihood of successful outcomes.

A critical component of any clinical trial is the monitoring of subjects, and AI has changed the stakes here too. With the use of smart collars and other wearable technology, real-time data collection has become feasible and valuable. These devices compile a continuous stream of information on vital signs, movement, and other health indicators. For researchers, this data provides granular insights, enabling more accurate assessments of a drug's efficacy and safety.

The analysis of this data was once a bottleneck in clinical trials. Traditional methods of data sorting and examination can be slow and cumbersome. Yet, AI-driven data analytics tools rapidly sift through mountains of information to identify patterns and anomalies. By using algorithms adept at recognizing trends across multidimensional datasets, researchers gain insights that were previously hard to detect. This analytical capability significantly accelerates the data evaluation phase, allowing veterinarians and researchers to draw conclusions with both speed and confidence.

Moreover, AI offers the potential to simulate clinical trials through computational models before any real-world implementation. Virtual trials, as they are known, allow researchers to test hypotheses and design protocols in a digital environment, refining their approaches based on the simulated outcomes. This preliminary work can drastically reduce the cost and risk associated with physical trials, leading to more focused and efficient execution when trials proceed with actual animal subjects.

The potential pitfalls of clinical trials, like unexpected side effects, are also mitigated with AI applications. Predictive models assist in foreseeing adverse reactions by cross-referencing new trial data with pre-existing drug response databases. This foresight not only protects animal welfare but also aids in refining treatment protocols, ensuring more targeted and humane approaches.

AI is not limited to just improving the trials themselves; it also impacts post-trial analysis and application. After a trial concludes, AI aids in the broader interpretation of results, crafting individualized patient care strategies based on trial data. This personalized approach marks a shift toward precision veterinary medicine, where findings from clinical trials directly inform tailored treatments for animals in the broader population.

Furthermore, the reach of AI-driven clinical trials isn't confined to domestic animals alone. Wildlife and exotic species, often underrepresented in traditional veterinary research, stand to benefit immensely. By utilizing AI to process complex ecological data, researchers can effectively conduct trials that inform conservation and rehabilitation efforts for endangered species with very specific medical and environmental needs.

Ethical considerations must evolve alongside this technological advancement. It's crucial that AI in clinical trials adheres to stringent ethical guidelines analogous to those in human medicine. Transparency in AI decision-making processes and adherence to animal welfare standards are paramount, ensuring that the benefits of AI do not overshadow the moral obligations inherent in veterinary care.

As AI continues to revolutionize clinical trials, the potential for collaborative advancements grows. Cross-disciplinary collaboration among veterinarians, AI experts, statisticians, and ethicists will pave the way for innovative solutions and set new standards for veterinary medicine. These partnerships are vital, turning AI from a powerful tool into an integral partner in solving some of veterinary medicine's most enduring challenges.

In summary, AI's transformative power in clinical trials lies in its ability to streamline processes, enhance the precision of results, and ultimately improve animal health care on a profound level. As the technology advances, its integration into veterinary clinical trials will not only continue to reshape the future but also to redefine the boundaries of what's possible in animal healthcare and conservation.

Chapter 6:
Telemedicine and AI

Telemedicine, once a futuristic concept, has become a reality, largely thanks to the integration of AI technologies in veterinary care. This leap forward allows for advanced remote diagnostics and consultations, breaking barriers that once constrained veterinary access to urban locales. AI algorithms enhance the ability to assess symptoms and provide accurate diagnoses from afar, making it possible for pet owners and veterinarians to connect over vast distances. Whether you're on a bustling farm or in a small city apartment, AI facilitates timely advice and intervention, promising a future where geographical boundaries no longer prevent animals from receiving prompt medical attention. Moreover, this expansion of telemedicine changes the dynamics of veterinary practice, offering a beacon of hope for reaching underserved areas and making quality care accessible to all. As AI continues to evolve, it holds the potential to reshape traditional approaches and open up new horizons in animal healthcare, empowering veterinarians and enhancing the lives of animals everywhere.

Remote Diagnoses and Consultations

As the digital landscape evolves, telemedicine in veterinary practice is undergoing a significant transformation, primarily driven by advances in artificial intelligence (AI). Remote diagnoses and consultations are creating new opportunities for veterinarians to extend their services beyond the physical walls of clinics. This shift is pivotal in reshaping the accessibility and quality of animal healthcare, allowing veterinarians to reach more patients and address medical concerns more promptly.

AI's capabilities open a new frontier in remote veterinary care, offering nuanced and comprehensive diagnostic tools that weren't possible just a few years ago. By analyzing vast datasets, machine learning algorithms can identify patterns and anomalies in animal health indicators that may elude even the most experienced eyes. This includes interpreting data from wearable devices, understanding complex imaging scans, or recognizing behavioral changes through video analysis.

The ability to consult a veterinarian from the comfort of home is transforming the way pet owners make decisions about their pet's health. During unexpected health concerns, these consultations provide immediate access to expertise without the stress of travel, particularly for anxious animals or those living in remote areas. AI enhances these interactions by offering veterinarians real-time data analysis and recommendations, granting a layer of insight that complements their professional judgment.

Moreover, AI-driven telemedicine platforms are breaking down geographic and logistical barriers, providing access to specialized veterinary care in regions where such services were previously limited or unavailable. By connecting veterinarians with specialists, pets now receive targeted advice and treatments that otherwise might have required long-distance travel. This exchange of expertise is crucial in cases where time and expertise are of the essence, such as rare diseases or complex surgical needs.

One of AI's most promising contributions to remote diagnostics is its ability to continually learn and improve its diagnostic acumen. Machine learning algorithms can be trained with an ever-expanding repository of veterinary cases, enhancing their ability to predict disease outcomes and suggest treatment plans. This means over time, these systems become even more accurate and comprehensive in their assessments.

Through telemedicine, AI also supports early disease detection and prevention strategies. By analyzing data from periodic remote consultations, AI can flag subtle signs of disease that may not warrant immediate concern but could evolve into something more severe if left unchecked. Early intervention, guided by AI insights, can significantly improve treatment success rates and animal welfare.

There's a synergistic potential that emerges when AI is integrated into telemedicine frameworks. While technology provides powerful tools for diagnosis and monitoring, the compassionate touch and nuanced judgment of veterinary professionals remain irreplaceable. Together, they create a robust system that ensures animals receive comprehensive care tailored to their unique circumstances.

Nevertheless, the integration of AI in telemedicine also presents challenges. Veterinarians and pet owners alike must navigate questions of data privacy and system accuracy, ensuring that AI aids are used ethically and responsibly. Establishing trust in these new technologies is paramount for successful adoption, and transparency in their application can help assuage concerns.

The financial implications of deploying AI in remote consultations are also significant. While initial investments may seem steep, the long-term benefits of streamlined operations, increased reach, and improved diagnostic accuracy promise returns that justify the expenditure. Furthermore, by optimizing resource allocation and reducing travel costs, veterinary practices can operate more efficiently, passing savings onto clients.

The growing prevalence of remote diagnoses accentuated by AI also brings about a necessary shift in the vet-client relationship. Clear communication becomes even more crucial in a virtual setting, where veterinarians must adeptly interpret AI analyses and convey accurate information in a reassuring manner. Training programs to support veterinarians in these new roles will be key to ensuring quality care remains consistent.

In summary, remote diagnoses and consultations facilitated by AI are revolutionizing veterinary medicine. They're expanding access, enhancing diagnostic accuracy, and fostering early intervention, ultimately setting a new standard for animal healthcare. Integrating these technologies thoughtfully ensures that veterinary professionals can harness their full potential, offering a new modality of care that is as compassionate as it is cutting-edge.

Expanding Access to Veterinary Care

Picture a world where veterinary care is accessible to every pet owner, regardless of geographic location or economic status. Thanks to telemedicine and artificial intelligence (AI), this vision is rapidly becoming a reality. The convergence of these technologies is reshaping the veterinary landscape, making high-quality animal care widely available and easy to access. By reducing barriers to care, AI and telemedicine have the potential to significantly broaden the reach of veterinary services, benefiting pets and their owners alike.

Telemedicine leverages digital communication tools, allowing veterinarians to consult with pet owners remotely. This innovation is not just convenient; it's a game-changer for those living in rural or underserved areas where veterinary clinics are often scarce or difficult to reach. Suddenly, pet owners no longer have to endure long journeys to the nearest veterinarian. Instead, a consultation can happen from the comfort of their home, saving time and simplifying logistics for both veterinarians and pet owners.

The incorporation of AI into telemedicine amplifies its advantages. AI helps triage cases, directing urgent issues to veterinarians while managing routine inquiries efficiently. The result is a streamlined process that saves valuable time and ensures that animals with the most critical needs receive attention first. AI can analyze symptoms and patterns in real-time, providing veterinarians with insightful data to inform their diagnoses. This swift and informed decision-making process enhances care quality and effectiveness.

Smaller practices may find it challenging to keep up with technological advancements. Here, AI and telemedicine offer a lifeline, equipping veterinarians with tools that would otherwise be financially out of reach. Access to AI-driven diagnostic tools and teleconsultations can level the playing field, ensuring smaller clinics can offer the same high standards of care as larger, more resource-rich establishments. This democratization of technology fosters a broader distribution of veterinary expertise, which is crucial in expanding accessibility.

Moreover, telemedicine and AI usher in a new level of convenience for pet owners. In the hustle and bustle of modern life, finding time for a vet visit can be daunting. Telemedicine removes the hassle of scheduling conflicts and travel, offering pet owners the flexibility they need. They can attend appointments outside regular office hours, enhancing accessibility for those constrained by work or personal commitments.

Financial considerations also play a significant role in expanding access to veterinary care. Traditional veterinary services often come with substantial costs, which can be prohibitive for some pet owners. By reducing overheads and improving efficiency, telemedicine and AI can lower the price of veterinary consultations, making them more attainable. This inclusivity not only helps individual pet owners but could also lead to earlier interventions and improved overall public health outcomes as more animals receive timely care.

On a larger scale, the integration of AI and telemedicine facilitates global collaboration among veterinary professionals. A veterinarian handling a challenging case in a remote region can easily connect with international experts, sharing knowledge and insights. This global network of real-time expertise sharing enriches the quality of care, transcending geographical and technological barriers. It propels the veterinary community toward a future where collaboration, rather than competition, drives progress and innovation.

Additionally, AI-supported systems can maintain comprehensive and accurate health records. Imagine a platform where a pet's health data is at the fingertips of any veterinarian who needs it, improving continuity and consistency of care. Such systems can enhance communication between pet owners and vets, providing reminders for vaccinations and check-ups, and ensuring no aspect of an animal's health is overlooked.

Despite these advancements, embracing telemedicine and AI isn't without challenges. Technology adoption requires training and a willingness to shift traditional practices. Veterinarians need to stay informed about emerging technologies and how to integrate them seamlessly into their operations. Overcoming these hurdles necessitates ongoing education and support, but the rewards are well worth the effort. By investing time and resources into understanding and utilizing these tools, veterinarians can open new avenues of care and support for their clients.

Furthermore, regulatory frameworks need to adapt to these innovations. Policies governing veterinary telemedicine must be continuously reviewed and updated to ensure they support the best practices in care while safeguarding privacy and ethical standards. Engaging with policymakers and regulatory bodies is crucial to forming an environment conducive to the growth of these technologies, fostering innovation while protecting consumers and animals.

The future of veterinary care hinges on embracing these technological shifts. As AI and telemedicine continue to evolve, the potential for further expanding access to veterinary services grows exponentially. The vision of comprehensive, compassionate, and universally accessible animal healthcare is no longer a distant dream, but an emerging reality. By continuing to adapt and integrate these technologies, veterinarians can not only enhance their practices but also improve the health and well-being of animals across the globe.

This promising synergy between AI and telemedicine is at the heart of modern veterinary medicine's evolution. As stewards of animal health, veterinarians are uniquely positioned to harness these tools, setting a new standard for accessibility and quality in care. With dedication, collaboration, and innovation, the field of veterinary medicine can transcend its current boundaries, providing exceptional care to every animal, everywhere.

Chapter 7:
AI for Exotic and Wildlife Care

The fusion of artificial intelligence and wildlife care is setting the stage for a new era of conservation and animal management. AI algorithms, combined with data from remote sensing technologies, are now capable of monitoring wildlife populations with precision and efficiency previously unimaginable. These advancements allow for real-time tracking of species, providing critical insights into migration patterns and habitat utilization. With AI's assistance, conservationists can make swift, data-driven decisions to protect endangered species and manage ecosystems sustainably. The integration of AI in these efforts is not only about conserving wildlife but also ensuring that biodiversity, a pivotal component of our planet's resilience, continues to thrive. By employing AI, we create a bridge between technology and nature, where the preservation of the wild becomes a shared responsibility between human innovation and the earth's natural wonders.

Monitoring Wildlife Populations

The natural world is vast and intricate, with millions of species interacting in complex ecosystems. Monitoring wildlife populations presents an intricate task requiring immense resources and dedication. However, artificial intelligence (AI) is increasingly playing a pivotal role in revolutionizing how we approach this challenge, offering unprecedented capabilities to observe, understand, and protect wildlife. As technological advances unfold, the potential for AI to contribute meaningfully to wildlife conservation becomes ever clearer.

To effectively monitor wildlife populations, accurate data collection and analysis are crucial. Traditionally, researchers relied heavily on manual data collection methods, which could be time-consuming, labor-intensive, and prone to human error. However, with AI, the game has changed. Machine learning algorithms can process vast amounts of data quickly and accurately, identifying patterns and providing insights that were previously unimaginable. For example, wildlife cameras equipped with AI can automatically identify species, count individuals, and even track movements without human intervention.

These AI-powered systems not only enhance accuracy but also expand the scale of monitoring projects. In remote areas like rainforests or across expansive savannahs, deploying networks of AI-enhanced sensors allows for continuous observations that aren't limited by human presence. Data collected in real-time is transmitted for immediate analysis, which is crucial for making timely conservation decisions. With AI, even the most inaccessible regions can become observable frontiers of biological inquiry.

Artificial intelligence also excels in processing satellite imagery and drone footage, unlocking new perspectives on wildlife populations and habitat changes. Sophisticated image recognition software can detect subtle environmental changes, such as deforestation or the expansion of human settlements, providing critical early warning signals of threats to wildlife habitats. These tools offer the promise of proactive conservation strategies, enabling swift actions to mitigate habitat degradation before it spirals out of control.

Furthermore, AI plays a key role in understanding wildlife behavior and migration patterns. By analyzing data from GPS collars or bio-logging devices, machine learning algorithms can track the movement and activities of animals with remarkable precision. This analysis can yield vital insights into migration routes, breeding grounds, and feeding habits, helping conservationists to secure critical habitats and corridors necessary for species survival. Respecting the balance of ecosystems, AI helps us become more effective stewards of natural resources.

One inspiring example of AI in action is the monitoring of endangered species like the African elephant. These majestic creatures face numerous threats from poaching to habitat loss. AI algorithms process data collected from aerial surveys and camera traps to estimate population sizes, detect poaching activities, and evaluate the effectiveness of protected areas. By leveraging AI, conservationists can save time and reduce costs, enabling them to allocate resources more strategically in the fight against extinction.

Intertwined with these technological advancements are ethical considerations regarding privacy and the potential impacts on local communities. While AI can bolster conservation, it is essential to ensure the data collection does not infringe on human rights or traditional knowledge systems. Incorporating local communities in AI-driven conservation efforts can foster collaboration, respect cultural heritage, and enhance the effectiveness of monitoring programs.

Integrating AI into wildlife monitoring also has repercussions for policy-making on conservation. Policymakers can leverage AI-generated data to create more informed and targeted conservation policies. For instance, when AI models predict potential human-wildlife conflict zones, authorities can develop strategies to minimize these encounters, benefiting both the wildlife and the local communities.

As we continue to harness AI in monitoring wildlife populations, the potential for innovation seems endless. The collaborative efforts between tech experts, wildlife biologists, and local communities have the unique opportunity to unveil new layers of understanding about our natural world. This cross-disciplinary approach can create a future where AI not only aids in preserving wildlife but partners with us in cultivating a sustainable coexistence with the planet's rich biodiversity.

In conclusion, the impact of AI on wildlife monitoring is profound. By enhancing our ability to observe and understand wildlife populations, AI empowers us to make informed decisions that can alter the course of conservation efforts worldwide. With continued research, development, and ethical consideration, AI stands to become a powerful ally in the global mission to protect and preserve the natural environment for generations to come. The future of wildlife conservation lies not only in understanding the threats these populations face but also in the innovative integration of technologies that help mitigate these challenges. AI represents a beacon of hope, heralding a new era of insight and action in biodiversity conservation.

AI in Conservation Efforts

As artificial intelligence continues to advance, its benefits are seeping into some of the most critical areas of environmental preservation. Wildlife conservation represents a groundbreaking domain where AI has a profound impact. Imagine having the ability to process vast amounts of data collected from various ecosystems worldwide. AI's involvement has opened new possibilities that were once just a part of a conservationist's dream. The role of AI in conservation efforts is multifaceted, encompassing species monitoring, habitat preservation, and poaching prevention, each contributing to the preservation of biodiversity.

One key application of AI in conservation is enhanced species monitoring. Historically, tracking wildlife has been labor-intensive, requiring practically living in the field to gather substantial data via sight and sound observations. Today, AI algorithms can process audio and visual feeds from cameras and microphones strategically deployed in the wild. By employing image recognition technologies, AI systems can identify and count specific animal species. This capability is crucial for tracking population dynamics and assessing the health of species in their natural habitats.

Not only do these advancements help save time and reduce human error, but they also provide real-time data. Conservationists can now make informed decisions swiftly, modulating their strategies based on current wildlife data rather than waiting months for it to be manually compiled and analyzed. For example, AI has been used to track the movements of the elusive snow leopard in Asia, providing critical data that helps formulate more effective conservation strategies.

In addition to monitoring species, AI plays a significant role in protecting habitats from degradation. AI-powered satellite imagery analysis can detect changes in land use, deforestation patterns, and climate-related impacts over large areas. These insights enable early intervention and help organizations direct their conservation efforts where they are needed most. By integrating predictive analytics, AI can also foresee potential habitat disruptions, providing a proactive approach to conservation.

Consider how AI can also assist in fighting illegal poaching—a persistent threat to wildlife globally. Poachers pose a significant risk to endangered species like elephants and rhinoceroses. To combat this, AI systems are now integrated with anti-poaching drones and sensors to monitor protected areas. These systems analyze movement patterns and can distinguish between human and non-human activities. On detecting suspicious movement, they alert rangers to potential poaching activities, giving them a leg up in intercepting illegal pursuits before they cause harm.

Furthermore, AI is playing a pivotal role in community-driven conservation efforts. Educating local communities and involving them in conservation work has been shown to yield positive outcomes. AI tools are employed to help convey complex data in understandable formats, thus fostering local engagement and empowerment. In regions where traditional conservation messaging has been less effective, AI-generated models and simulations bring compelling narratives to life, promoting considerations of sustainability among local stakeholders.

The conservation efforts assisted by AI are not limited to land. Marine conservation has also seen breakthroughs with AI applications. Ocean ecosystems are delicate and often out of sight, making monitoring and preservation challenging. AI systems, however, are enhancing how we track ocean health and marine life. By analyzing patterns from satellite data, ocean sensors, and automated underwater vehicles, AI models predict the impacts of climate phenomena, assess coral reef health, and map the distribution of fish populations, aiding conservation in these vast, underwater expanses.

An exciting facet of AI-driven conservation is its predictive capabilities. AI thrives on patterns and probabilities, allowing conservationists to anticipate trends in animal behavior and environmental changes. By simulating various scenarios, AI helps manage resources more effectively, cater to sudden environmental changes, and ensure that the necessary actions are taken to prevent wildlife crises.

Collaboration between technologists and conservationists is crucial for unlocking AI's full potential in wildlife conservation. Through effective partnerships, AI tools are crafted to address real-world conservation challenges, ensuring that technology and ecological knowledge synergize seamlessly. Additionally, interdisciplinary initiatives are fostering innovation, creating an integrated approach to conservation efforts that leverage AI's capabilities comprehensively.

Finally, the successful integration of AI into conservation strategy must be complemented by ethical considerations. Ensuring that AI applications do not inadvertently harm ecosystems is essential. Conservationists must remain vigilant against data misuse or technology-driven disturbances in wildlife habitats, and efforts must abide by ecological ethics and data privacy considerations.

In conclusion, AI offers a transformative toolkit in our efforts to conserve the world's precious, yet fragile, ecosystems. The potential of AI to revolutionize how we approach conservation is both inspiring and motivational. As we advance, AI becomes an ally in overcoming the seemingly insurmountable challenges faced in conservation work. With technology on our side, a future of flourishing biodiversity no longer feels out of reach.

Chapter 8:
Predictive Analytics in Animal Health

Predictive analytics is transforming the landscape of animal healthcare by leveraging the power of AI to foresee health trends and enable proactive management. Veterinarians are now able to tap into vast datasets, uncovering patterns and anomalies that were previously invisible. This technological leap allows practitioners to anticipate diseases before they manifest visibly, providing a significant edge in preventive care. By analyzing behavioral and physiological data collected from a variety of species, predictive models can pinpoint potential health risks, leading to interventions that safeguard animal well-being. Think of it as a guardian angel for our animal companions, ensuring their health is maintained with foresight. The integration of predictive analytics not only enhances decision-making but also fosters a deeper understanding of complex health dynamics. As we look to the future, the continued evolution of these analytics will no doubt usher in a new era of animal care driven by data, empathy, and precision.

Forecasting Health Trends

In the rapidly evolving landscape of veterinary medicine, the ability to anticipate future health trends stands as a game-changer, empowered by the enhancements brought about by predictive analytics. Predictive analytics in animal health leverages historical and real-time data, utilizes complex algorithms, and applies sophisticated modeling to foresee future health outcomes. This capability enables veterinarians to make informed decisions that improve the quality and efficiency of animal healthcare.

At the heart of this transformation is the wealth of data available from various sources, such as electronic health records, wearable tech, and environmental monitoring systems. By harnessing the analytical power of AI, veterinarians can identify patterns and trends that were previously buried in immense datasets. These insights become pivotal in predicting potential health issues, identifying at-risk populations, and even catching the early signs of emerging diseases.

Consider the implications of this technology in managing infectious diseases among animal populations. Predictive analytics allows for the analysis of geographical and temporal patterns of disease spread, identifying potential outbreaks before they occur. This proactive stance enables timely interventions, potentially averting large-scale disease outbreaks that can have devastating effects on livestock and wildlife. Early identification and containment of disease not only save lives but also reduce economic losses associated with livestock disease management.

Another significant area within forecasting health trends is recognizing the onset of chronic conditions in pets. Chronic illnesses like diabetes, renal failure, and arthritis can be diagnosed earlier with the help of AI by identifying subtle changes in behavior or biological markers over time. By foreseeing these conditions, treatment plans can be adjusted promptly, improving the quality of life for our animal companions and potentially increasing their lifespan.

The scope of predictive analytics extends beyond individual cases to broader public health issues. Veterinary public health is underscored by the need to monitor zoonotic diseases—those that can be transmitted from animals to humans. AI-driven predictive models can play a crucial role in understanding and controlling zoonotic outbreaks, offering significant benefits to both animal and human health sectors.

Additionally, climate change plays a role in shifting health trends that affect animal populations globally. Variables such as temperature changes, migration patterns, and food availability directly impact animal health, influencing disease vectors and habitat conditions. AI analytics can synthesize environmental data with health metrics to predict challenges and guide adaptive management strategies in wildlife conservation and domestic animal welfare.

As veterinarians and tech enthusiasts delve deeper into forecasting health trends using AI, they must also navigate challenges such as data privacy, accuracy of predictions, and integration of AI into existing veterinary systems. The precision of models hinges on the quality of input data. Therefore, ensuring comprehensive data collection and addressing potential biases become critical tasks to achieve reliable forecasts.

Training in the interpretation of AI outputs is also pertinent. Veterinarians must be equipped to understand and apply these insights effectively. Collaboration between AI experts and veterinary professionals is necessary to bridge the gap between technological possibilities and practical application in everyday veterinary practice.

By optimizing forecasting capabilities, veterinary practices can shift from a reactive approach to a proactive one, characterized by preemptive health management. This transformation aligns with the overarching goal of AI in animal health—to elevate care through anticipatory, tailored interventions that foster better health outcomes for animals. As AI continues to evolve, its potential to revolutionize veterinary medicine promises a future where health issues are anticipated and mitigated before they escalate, ensuring the well-being of animals around the world.

Proactive Health Management

In the realm of veterinary medicine, predictive analytics is revolutionizing how we manage animal health. The concept of proactive health management is at the forefront of this transformation. By using data-driven predictions, veterinarians can anticipate potential health issues before they become critical, allowing for preemptive actions that can save lives, reduce costs, and improve the overall wellbeing of animals.

Proactive health management is not just a futuristic fantasy; it's rapidly becoming a reality thanks to advancements in AI technologies. By harnessing the power of predictive analytics, veterinarians can move beyond reactive care—where actions are taken after symptoms arise— to a model that emphasizes prevention and early intervention. This fundamental shift in approach promises to enhance the quality of care and extend the lifespan of animals by addressing health concerns at their nascent stages.

One of the hallmark applications of proactive health management is in disease prevention. With predictive analytics, veterinarians can analyze historical and real-time health data to identify patterns that might signal emerging health concerns. This approach is akin to anticipating the next move in a chess game; by anticipating patterns, veterinarians can make informed decisions that alter the course of an animal's health journey before problems manifest in clinical symptoms.

Moreover, predictive analytics enables the early detection of genetic disorders. By analyzing an animal's genetic makeup alongside prevalence data of certain conditions within breeds or species, veterinarians can offer insights into predispositions for specific diseases. This knowledge allows animal caretakers to take preemptive steps through customized care plans, potentially incorporating lifestyle adjustments and regular monitoring to stave off the development of these ailments.

Vaccination strategies can also benefit significantly from proactive health management. Traditionally, vaccination schedules are based on generalized timelines and often rely on retrospective disease outbreak data. However, by implementing predictive analytics, veterinarians can devise vaccination plans that are more targeted and responsive to actual risk levels. This way, animals receive vaccinations specifically tailored to anticipated exposures, maximizing efficacy while minimizing unnecessary interventions.

In companion animals, predictive modeling can address chronic conditions like obesity and diabetes. By evaluating lifestyle data, such as diet and exercise patterns, alongside health metrics, veterinarians can foresee potential issues. Recommendations for dietary changes or exercise routines can be proactively made, preventing the onset of related health problems. It's about catching the drift of the problem before the wave hits shore, ensuring animals maintain optimum health throughout their lives.

A paradigm shift is also evident in parasite management. With climate change affecting the distribution and prevalence of ecto- and endoparasites, predictive analytics aids veterinarians by predicting potential infestation peaks and advising timely interventions. This approach extends beyond mere treatment to encompass preventive care, formulating action plans that safeguard animal health proactively, mitigating infestations before they become widespread.

The integration of wearable technology further bolsters proactive health management. These devices continuously collect vital data regarding an animal's health, including heart rate, activity levels, and body temperature. By feeding this data into predictive models, veterinarians and pet owners receive timely alerts on irregularities, enabling swift action. This constant stream of information transforms the way health is monitored, making traditional periodic check-ups a complement to rather than the core of health surveillance.

Livestock management stands to gain tremendously from these advancements. In agricultural settings, where the health of large animal populations must be managed efficiently, predictive analytics offer unparalleled insights into herd health dynamics. Farmers can predict and prevent outbreaks of infectious diseases, maintain productivity levels, and ensure food safety by understanding health trends and implementing tailored interventions. Essentially, it's precision agriculture with a health-centric focus.

As AI technologies become more sophisticated, the scope and accuracy of predictive models will only improve. Enhanced algorithms will better handle multifaceted datasets, providing even deeper insights into the health status of animals. Innovations such as deep learning may allow for the interpretation of complex interactions among diverse health indicators, making predictive health management progressively more reliable and robust.

Nevertheless, successful implementation of proactive health management requires collaboration and education. Veterinarians and researchers must work hand-in-hand to ensure algorithms are fed quality data and that predictions align with clinical realities. Additionally, educating pet owners, farmers, and zoo caretakers about these technological advancements will foster trust and acceptance, allowing for a smoother transition to this new era of veterinary care.

Ultimately, proactive health management represents a paradigm shift in veterinary medicine. It's a powerful reminder that the future of animal care lies in anticipation, not reaction. By focusing efforts upstream, addressing potential health issues before they become crises, we craft a narrative for animal health that doesn't just respond to challenges but actively shapes a healthier future. The sight of this horizon should inspire every veterinarian, animal lover, and tech enthusiast about the potential to transform animal healthcare holistically.

Chapter 9:
AI in Nutrition and Diet Planning

In the realm of veterinary medicine, the integration of AI into nutrition and diet planning marks a revolutionary advancement, promising customized health solutions for our animal companions. Harnessing vast datasets, AI algorithms can assess specific nutritional needs and craft precise diet plans tailored to each animal's unique physiology and lifestyle. This personalization goes beyond traditional methods, offering insights that were once unachievable. AI-driven tools meticulously monitor dietary intake and adjust nutritional strategies in real-time, ensuring optimal health and performance. This dynamic approach revitalizes animal care, moving it toward preventive measures rather than reactive ones, and ultimately improving the quality of life for countless creatures. Through technology's lens, veterinarians can now advocate for diets that consider immediate demands and adapt to future challenges, paving the way for robust animal wellness.

Custom Diets for Optimal Health

In a world where precision is the forefront in the veterinary sphere, custom diets powered by artificial intelligence are redefining optimal health for animals. Recent advancements in AI provide an unprecedented opportunity to tailor nutrition plans that are finely tuned to each animal's unique dietary needs, taking into account species, breed, age, activity level, health status, and even genetic background. No longer are we relying solely on broad-based dietary solutions; instead, we are embracing a future where each pet and farm animal can benefit from dining like a connoisseur while still meeting every dietary requirement.

Artificial intelligence, with its ability to process vast amounts of data, is revolutionizing the way veterinarians and nutritionists approach animal diets. By analyzing extensive datasets, AI systems identify nutritional trends and deficiencies that would be impossible to discern otherwise. This not only ensures that diets are nutritionally complete but also optimizes the health outcomes for each animal. With AI, the mantra "you are what you eat" evolves into a scientific maxim — one grounded in data-driven customization.

Consider the complexities that pet owners face today: the shelves filled with an overwhelming array of pet food options and the nuanced needs of different breeds or health conditions. It's a daunting task to distinguish which diets might reduce inflammation, support cognitive function, or bolster immunity. With AI, these decisions transform from guesswork into an evidence-based process, offering owners peace of mind. Intelligent diet planning tools leverage data from thousands of cases worldwide, allowing for dietary solutions that are tried, tested, and true.

AI's capabilities don't end at diet creation. Nutritional monitoring technologies are being embedded transparently into smart collars and devices, constantly collecting data on an animal's health metrics. These devices transmit real-time insights back to dietary management systems, crafting an ongoing dialogue between what an animal eats and its overall health. Any alterations in weight, digestion, or energy levels can instantly prompt adjustments within the diet plan to better align with the animal's current needs, thereby holding the key to dynamic nutrition.

Moreover, AI's role in custom diets stretches beyond individual pets and touches the agricultural spectrum. Livestock farming benefits enormously from predictive dietary planning, which can improve growth rates and enhance meat or milk quality while considering environmental sustainability. With AI, the feed for livestock can be optimized to not only focus on growth and productivity but also on reducing the carbon footprint, an increasingly crucial consideration in today's environmentally-conscious world.

On another front, tailored diets can also play a vital role in healthcare management strategies for animals with chronic diseases. Animals suffering from ailments like diabetes, kidney problems, or obesity require stringent dietary regimens. AI can calculate precisely what these animals need and can provide alert systems to notify veterinarians and pet owners of necessary changes. Additionally, personalized diet plans enhance the efficacy of medical treatments by ensuring that nutrient intake supports prescribed therapies.

What sets AI apart is its capacity for learning and adaptation. As more data pours in, AI systems continually refine their recommendations, making every successive diet plan more precise than the last. It's a cycle of perpetual improvement where AI learns from each dietary tweak, success, and even failure, turning static recipes into dynamic, living guides for optimal nutrition.

Indeed, while AI presents cutting-edge solutions, its integration into routine practice requires collaboration among veterinarians, AI experts, and pet owners. As these parties join forces, they must navigate the delicate balance between technology and care, ensuring that data-driven insights never overshadow the individual or emotional needs of the animals. The human touch remains indispensable in this innovative process. Veterinarians, with their unique understanding of animal behavior and history, will always be integral to interpreting AI's outputs and conveying them in empathetic, actionable therapies for owners.

The road ahead for custom diets in AI is brimming with potential, promising to address many of the world's ongoing nutritional challenges in the animal kingdom. As AI continues to map and model the biochemical nuances of different species, we edge closer to understanding and implementing diets that not only meet physiological needs but accelerate wellness and longevity.

In conclusion, AI's application in creating customized diets is more than just about meeting nutritional needs; it's about pioneering a future where animals thrive on truly personalized nutrition. This is a future where every meal is a step towards better health, where diet becomes an active, evolving partner in the wellness journey of each animal. With relentless innovation and collaboration, AI is turning this vision into reality, fueling the hopes of a healthier world for all creatures, great and small.

Nutritional Monitoring Technologies

In the realm of veterinary medicine, nutrition is the bedrock of animal health, playing a crucial role in both prevention and treatment of diseases. With the surge in AI technologies, nutritional monitoring for animals has undergone a remarkable transformation. The marriage of AI with diet planning is revolutionizing how veterinarians approach dietary interventions, ensuring tailored and precise nutritional guidance that is both proactive and reactive.

At the heart of this transformation is the use of advanced sensors and wearable devices designed to monitor an animal's nutritional intake and overall health metrics in real time. These devices collect data on various parameters such as food consumption, activity levels, and even biometric indicators like heart rate and temperature. This sea of data is then crunched by AI algorithms to provide veterinarians with distilled insights that can drive better dietary decisions.

One of the game-changers in this field is the ability of AI-driven platforms to create personalized diet plans. These plans don't just consider the animal's species, age, and weight, but also delve into more nuanced factors like genetic disposition, past health records, and even lifestyle factors specific to each animal. The result is a nutritional blueprint that aims to optimize health outcomes by preemptively addressing potential health issues related to diet.

Moreover, AI in nutritional monitoring isn't just about responding to data but about learning from it. Machine learning algorithms employed in these systems improve over time, learning patterns from the collected data that may not be immediately obvious to human eyes. For example, subtle changes in an animal's eating habits might predict an impending health issue, allowing veterinarians to intervene before a problem manifests.

Furthermore, predictive analytics play a pivotal role in the nutritional landscape. They're employed to forecast nutritional deficiencies or excesses that could lead to health complications. This proactive approach allows for adjustments to be made in dietary plans before symptoms emerge, effectively preventing issues like obesity, malnutrition, or metabolic diseases.

In addition to preventive care, AI technologies offer invaluable support in managing chronic conditions. For instance, animals suffering from diabetes or kidney disease require meticulous monitoring of their diet. Here, AI technologies can assist by analyzing real-time data and adjusting dietary recommendations instantaneously to keep the animal's condition in check.

Particularly exciting is the level of granularity that these AI systems can offer. They can parse through a spectrum of dietary components—proteins, fats, carbohydrates—and evaluate their effects on an animal's physiology with considerable precision. By doing so, veterinarians are better equipped to recommend specific dietary adjustments that cater to individual health needs, potentially increasing the efficacy of treatments and ongoing health support.

The integration of AI-driven nutritional monitoring is not without its challenges, however. These sophisticated systems require rigorous validation and verification to ensure accuracy and reliability in their recommendations. Data privacy and the ethical implications of continuous monitoring are additional concerns that need addressing as these technologies proliferate.

Despite these hurdles, the adoption of AI in nutrition is steadily increasing, with veterinary practitioners reporting enhanced outcomes in both preventive and therapeutic nutrition management. Animals are now receiving diet-based interventions that are as unique as their own paw prints, reflecting the deep understanding AI applications have brought into this sphere of veterinary medicine.

As we look ahead, the potential for AI to predict optimal feeding times, determine ideal nutrient combinations, and even suggest lifestyle changes tailored to the animal's evolving needs is tantalizing. These advancements promise a future where animal nutrition is not just about feeding but about strategic nurturing of health and wellbeing, solidifying AI's role as an indispensable ally in animal healthcare.

Chapter 10:
Smart Technology in Animal Monitoring

Imagine a world where animals communicate their health status through intelligent devices, creating seamless connections between their well-being and veterinary care. This is not science fiction. With the integration of smart technology in animal monitoring, veterinarians now have unprecedented tools at their disposal to observe and understand animal health in real-time. Wearable devices for animals, equipped with sensors and GPS, are leading this technological revolution. These gadgets collect a treasure trove of data—from heart rate and activity levels to precise locations—making health tracking more thorough and immediate. Such real-time insights allow for timely interventions and enhanced care, transforming how professionals approach animal health management. This technological leap doesn't just bring innovation; it inspires a new level of engagement and empathy in veterinary practices, ensuring animals receive the proactive and personalized care they deserve. As we navigate these advancements, we're not only revolutionizing animal healthcare but also enhancing the bond we share with our animal companions.

Wearable Devices for Animals

Wearable technology isn't just changing how humans monitor their health; it's reshaping how we care for animals too. As AI continues to evolve, this synergy between tech and veterinary medicine offers compelling possibilities. From fitness trackers to smart collars, these devices collect valuable data, helping pet owners and veterinarians stay on top of an animal's well-being.

Today, wearable devices for animals cover a wide range of functionalities. Imagine a collar that monitors not just a dog's location, but also tracks heart rate, body temperature, and sleep patterns. These devices can send alerts when anomalies are detected, enabling early interventions. The data collected is pivotal for observing long-term health trends, offering insights that were previously difficult to obtain.

For livestock, wearable tech isn't just a fancy gadget but a revolution in farm management. Understanding the health metrics of an entire herd in real-time can prevent outbreaks of diseases and improve overall farm productivity. Temperature sensors and GPS trackers can help farmers make data-driven decisions about their cattle's health and grazing patterns. This blend of AI and wearable technology promises to optimize agricultural practices while ensuring animal health is not compromised.

Now, one might wonder, how do these devices actually work? Most wearable devices for animals are equipped with sensors that capture various health metrics. These metrics are processed using advanced algorithms to deliver actionable insights. For instance, if a horse isn't moving as much as it normally does, the device can alert the owner, who might then investigate a potential injury or illness sooner, rather than later.

Behavioral monitoring is yet another groundbreaking application of wearable tech. Cats, being notorious for masking symptoms, can benefit immensely from smart collars that track activity levels and provide data to ascertain the feline's health changes over time. Pet owners find solace in knowing they have a window into the less obvious signs of distress or illness.

The integration of AI with wearable devices becomes particularly powerful when we consider customization. Each animal is unique, and these devices can be tailored to suit specific needs. Machine learning algorithms analyze data over time, learning what 'normal' looks like for each animal and flagging deviations that might indicate health issues.

Moreover, veterinary practices are increasingly focusing on preventive care. With the help of wearables, veterinarians can prescribe and monitor fitness regimes or dietary plans, providing a holistic approach to animal care. The ability to gather continuous health data empowers professionals to make well-informed decisions that enhance the quality of life for animals.

A challenge that both developers and users face is ensuring comfort and practicality. Animals, much like humans, must find these devices non-intrusive. Innovations are constantly being made to make devices smarter, lighter, and adaptable for various species and sizes. Ensuring seamless integration into their daily lives without causing distress is paramount.

Cost, too, has historically been a barrier to widespread adoption. However, as technology advances, the affordability of these devices is improving. This democratization of smart tech allows more pet owners and veterinarians access to advanced monitoring solutions. As costs decrease, the potential benefits expand exponentially, reaching into homes, farms, and even wildlife settings.

Speaking of wildlife, conservationists are utilizing this tech to track migrations, monitor at-risk species, and study behavior under changing climates. Non-invasive devices gather crucial ecological data, bolstering efforts to understand and protect the animal kingdom comprehensively. With climate change and habitat destruction looming, this technology could not be more timely.

Importantly, the data collected by these devices also enriches research databases, pushing the boundaries of veterinary medicine. Through AI-driven analysis of large datasets, we can derive patterns and predictions previously impossible to achieve. This insight propels research, opening doors to early disease detection and novel treatment approaches.

The future holds endless possibilities. The fusion of AI and wearable technology seems destined to become the new norm in animal healthcare, continually evolving with innovation. As this field grows, so does our ability to provide better and more individualized care for creatures great and small.

In conclusion, wearable devices for animals are not just about technology; they're about bridges—connecting us more intimately with our animal companions. They redefine animal care, offering a glimpse into a future where health monitoring is not only sophisticated but proactive. This synergy between technology and empathy is likely to lead to healthier, happier lives for animals around the world.

Real-Time Health Tracking

The dynamic landscape of veterinary medicine is witnessing a transformative wave, propelled by the infusion of smart technology with real-time health tracking capabilities. This innovation stands at the forefront of revolutionizing how veterinarians monitor and respond to animal health needs. By blending advanced sensors and data analytics, real-time health tracking is breathing new life into traditional animal monitoring methods, offering unprecedented insights into an animal's well-being.

In a world where time is of the essence, particularly when it comes to health, the ability to track an animal's condition in real time presents a significant leap forward. Sensors embedded in wearable devices can continuously monitor various health parameters, such as heart rate, temperature, and activity levels, transmitting this data to veterinary professionals instantly. These devices alert veterinarians to abnormalities before they escalate into serious health issues, facilitating early intervention and potentially saving lives.

Wearable technology tailored for animals is an intricate blend of engineering and design. Devices such as smart collars and biosensors have become increasingly sophisticated, offering more than just basic location tracking. For instance, the data harnessed from a wearable can provide a comprehensive picture of an animal's physical activity, its resting periods, and even signs of stress or discomfort. With the integration of AI analytics, these datasets can be synthesized, offering predictive insights into health trajectories.

One of the most profound impacts of real-time health tracking is its potential for preventive care. By readily capturing changes in normal behaviors, anomalies can be flagged for further investigation. This early detection plays a crucial role in preventing the development of chronic conditions. For example, subtle variations in a dog's activity pattern could signal the onset of arthritis, allowing for timely therapeutic interventions that can improve or maintain quality of life.

Moreover, real-time monitoring offers significant advantages in managing chronic conditions. Animals with chronic illnesses require consistent care and attention, often involving regular vet visits and detailed care plans. Real-time health tracking minimizes guesswork, as continuous data collection provides veterinarians with precise information regarding treatment efficacy and disease progression. Adjustments to treatment plans can be swiftly implemented based on the objective data collected from these devices.

Veterinarians are not the sole beneficiaries of this technological advancement. Pet owners themselves are empowered by having direct access to their pets' health data. This fosters a collaborative caregiver dynamic, where owners can engage proactively with their pets' health management. Having insights into their animal's well-being allows owners to make informed decisions and respond to potential issues quickly, reducing anxiety and enhancing the care experience.

Beyond the realm of domestic pets, real-time health tracking is significantly altering the landscape of wildlife conservation efforts. The ability to monitor animals in their natural habitats without intrusive methods offers invaluable data for research purposes. This technology enables scientists to track migration patterns, monitor the health of endangered species, and better understand ecological impacts on wildlife health.

The transformative potential of real-time health tracking can also be seen in farm management. Livestock health is crucial to agricultural productivity, and smart technology facilitates more effective monitoring of herds. For instance, wearable devices can provide data on an animal's eating habits and detect signs of illness early on, helping to prevent the spread of disease and maintaining herd health. This not only enhances welfare but also ensures economic viability for farmers.

Real-time health tracking is redefining the scale and scope of veterinary care. As algorithms grow more sophisticated, they promise to not only interpret data with accuracy but to also learn from patterns and experience. This continuous loop of feedback and refinement heralds a future where the predictive capacity of AI in animal health monitoring reaches its zenith, potentially transforming the very practice of veterinary medicine.

However, with great innovation comes challenges. Data privacy and security remain paramount concerns in the deployment of real-time health tracking technologies. As vast amounts of data are collected and transmitted, ensuring that this information is safeguarded against breaches is crucial. Veterinarians and tech developers must collaborate to establish rigorous standards to protect the integrity and confidentiality of health data.

Furthermore, the integration of these technologies into everyday veterinary practice demands a shift in mindset. It requires both veterinarians and pet owners to engage in continuous learning about the capabilities and limitations of real-time tracking systems. Education becomes a vital tool in overcoming resistance, inspiring confidence in the technology's ability to complement rather than replace traditional veterinary wisdom.

The road ahead is filled with possibilities, as real-time health tracking technologies become more accessible and affordable. With ongoing advancements, the barriers to their adoption will diminish, paving the way for widespread implementation across diverse veterinary settings. This technological embrace promises to enhance animal health outcomes and elevate the standard of care, inviting veterinary professionals to reimagine how they approach diagnostics, treatment, and long-term animal welfare.

Ultimately, real-time health tracking stands as a testament to the incredible synergy possible between technology and compassionate animal care. By leveraging the power of real-time data, we move closer to a future where health monitoring is not just reactive but anticipates needs, aligning with the core mission of enhancing animal well-being. The horizon is bright with potential, and the journey towards integrated smart technology in veterinary care is only just beginning.

Chapter 11:
AI in Behavior Analysis

Artificial Intelligence is starting to reshape how we understand and manage animal behavior, offering promising possibilities for veterinarians and animal caretakers alike. By harnessing vast datasets and advanced algorithms, AI systems can analyze subtle patterns in animal behavior that might elude human observation. These insights are invaluable in addressing behavioral issues early and tailoring interventions that improve animal welfare. In a world where the nuances of animal communication are complex, AI acts as a bridge, translating behaviors into actionable data. This strategic application not only enhances the quality of care animals receive but also offers a richer understanding of their unique needs and environmental interactions. As AI continues to evolve, its potential to transform our bond with animals grows exponentially, inspiring a future where technology and empathy work hand in hand.

Understanding Animal Behavior

Animal behavior often seems like an enigma, a complex dance of instinct and interaction. For centuries, humans have tried to decipher the ways animals communicate, their social structures, and their response to changing environments. In veterinary medicine, understanding animal behavior is crucial—not only for providing the right care but also for ensuring that animals and humans coexist harmoniously. With the rise of artificial intelligence, the way we analyze and interpret these behaviors is undergoing a revolutionary shift.

AI has set foot into realms previously reserved for intuition and experiential knowledge. The key to this entrance lies in its capability to process vast amounts of data far beyond human ability. By analyzing video footage, physiological signals, and environmental data, AI can discern patterns and anomalies in animal behavior that might escape even the most trained eye. This capability isn't merely about spotting oddities; it's about forming a deep, predictive understanding that can revolutionize animal care.

Imagine a scenario where a subtle change in an animal's routine can be detected before it leads to stress or illness. AI systems, equipped with sophisticated algorithms, can predict these shifts by evaluating behavioral data. For instance, a dog that paces more than usual might be experiencing anxiety, while a drop in activity for a typically energetic cat could signal illness. These insights are invaluable, allowing caregivers to intervene early, potentially preventing more serious health issues.

The potential of AI in behavior analysis extends to various species, from common household pets to exotic animals. Elephants in a sanctuary might exhibit certain behaviors that suggest stress, which could be related to environmental changes. With AI, conservationists and veterinarians can identify these stressors more accurately, making it possible to adjust conditions to better support the animals' well-being.

Additionally, AI is proving transformative in studying complex social structures among species. For example, in a herd of goats, certain individuals may exhibit behaviors indicating hierarchical changes or health issues. Machine learning models can analyze these interactions, providing insights into social dynamics that were once the domain of long-term observational studies. These insights not only aid in the immediate management of animal groups but can inform breeding and conservation strategies over the long term.

The application of AI doesn't stop at observation. It provides a robust framework for addressing behavioral issues that might arise in captive settings or among domestic animals. One significant area is in training and rehabilitating animals. Using AI, veterinarians and animal behaviorists can develop personalized training regimens based on the individual behavioral profiles of animals. This customization leads to more effective interventions and a higher likelihood of overcoming behavioral challenges.

AI's role in understanding animal behavior also dovetails with its applications in personalized treatments and nutritional planning, as covered in other chapters. By recognizing behavioral cues linked to dietary preferences or medical needs, tailored interventions can be designed that promote better health and quality of life for animals. The integration of AI in these domains highlights the interconnectivity of health and behavior, reinforcing the importance of a holistic approach to animal care.

Despite these advancements, the integration of AI into behavior analysis isn't without its challenges. One of the primary concerns is ensuring that AI systems operate ethically and enhance, rather than detract from, the human-animal bond. The data-driven insights from AI must be used to support empathetic care, emphasizing compassion alongside technological innovation.

Moreover, the success of AI in understanding animal behavior relies heavily on the quality of data and the intellectual synergy between AI experts and veterinarians. Collaboration is key, as outlined in later chapters, to develop models that truly reflect the multifaceted nature of animal behavior. This partnership ensures that AI tools are designed with a genuine understanding of animal welfare at their core.

Looking to the future, the potential for AI in animal behavior analysis appears limitless. As technology evolves, so too will our methods for not only interpreting animal behavior but predicting it. This predictive power could offer unprecedented levels of foresight, allowing veterinarians and caregivers to preemptively address issues before they manifest fully. Such advancements hold the promise of enhanced animal welfare across various contexts and species.

In conclusion, AI is a powerful ally in our quest to understand animal behavior. By harnessing its capabilities, we can achieve a deeper comprehension of the animals we care for and share our world with. This leap forward in understanding empowers veterinarians, enhances animal welfare, and ultimately, fosters a greater appreciation and respect for the rich tapestry of life behaviors around us.

Addressing Behavioral Issues

Addressing behavioral issues in animals is no small feat. It requires not only a deep understanding of animal psychology but also a keen observation of their interactions and environments. With the advancement of artificial intelligence, we have new tools at our disposal that can revolutionize this area of veterinary care. AI offers a lens through which we can dissect and comprehend the intricacies of behavior—whether it's a household pet exhibiting signs of stress or a wild animal adapting to a shrinking habitat. But how exactly does AI step in to address these challenges?

The first step in addressing behavioral issues is identifying the underlying causes. AI systems can sift through vast amounts of data, analyzing patterns that might elude even the most trained eyes. For instance, through video analysis, AI can detect subtle changes in an animal's gait or posture that could indicate discomfort or anxiety. These insights are particularly invaluable for animals who cannot easily express their distress through vocalization, such as fish or reptiles. By understanding these silent signals, veterinarians can intervene at the right moment, preventing small issues from escalating into more significant problems.

Moreover, AI-driven behavior analysis isn't only about spotting problems; it's about predicting them. Algorithms that analyze historical behavior data can flag potential future issues, allowing for proactive measures. This predictive power transforms the way we approach animal behavior. It lets us move from a reactive stance—only addressing problems when they become apparent—to a proactive one, where potential issues are anticipated and managed before they manifest. Imagine the relief for pet owners knowing that their dog's increasing restlessness during stormy weather has been predicted well in advance, giving them time to implement calming strategies.

In the veterinary field, behavioral assessments often rely on subjective judgment, which can vary from one practitioner to another. AI can bring a layer of objectivity to these assessments. Through machine learning, AI systems can be trained to cluster behavioral data into recognizable categories, aiding vets in distinguishing between normal eccentricities and behaviors that warrant further examination. For instance, AI can help determine if a cat's excessive grooming is a routine behavior for stress relief or a signal of a dermatological issue. This capacity for nuanced analysis enhances diagnostic accuracy and ensures that animals receive the most appropriate care.

One of the more exciting developments in AI-enhanced behavior analysis is the use of natural language processing (NLP). While animals don't speak human languages, they do communicate in their way. NLP can be used to analyze vocalizations or other sound patterns to interpret mood states or intentions. For example, in wildlife conservation, understanding the vocalizations of specific species can alert researchers to changes in environment or stress levels, elements that are crucial for preservation efforts. This technology bridges the gap between humans and animals, offering a more comprehensive understanding of animal welfare needs.

Another critical area where AI is making a difference is in the design of enriching environments. Behavioral problems often stem from inadequate stimulation or improper environments. AI can model optimal living conditions, suggesting changes that might improve an animal's well-being. Whether it's advising modifications in a zoo exhibit to encourage natural behaviors or recommending changes in the layout of a pet's living space, AI can create environments that better meet the physiological and psychological needs of animals. This creates a virtuous cycle: healthier environments lead to healthier behaviors, which in turn demand less intervention.

Wearable technology also plays a pivotal role in addressing behavioral issues, and AI enhances its capabilities significantly. Sensors on collars or harnesses can provide continuous data on activity levels, heart rates, and more. AI analyzes this information in real-time, providing insights into stress levels, exercise needs, or social interactions. The continuous monitoring allows for instant feedback and adjustment, facilitating quicker responses to anomalous behavior. Such data-driven insights equip veterinarians and pet owners alike with a powerful toolkit to ensure animals lead balanced lives.

Despite these advancements, challenges do arise. AI systems must be trained on diverse datasets to avoid biases that could skew analysis, especially in species or breeds that differ markedly in behavior. Collaboration between AI developers and veterinary professionals is essential to ensure these systems are robust and reliable. Moreover, ethical considerations must guide AI implementation, ensuring that interventions respect and support the natural behaviors and welfare of animals.

Finally, integration of AI in addressing behavioral issues holds the promise of broad accessibility. Not every pet owner has state-of-the-art behavioral clinics nearby, yet through AI solutions—many of which can be accessed via smartphones or consumer-grade devices—insights are readily available to a wider audience. This democratization of animal behavioral science ensures that more animals benefit from high-quality, informed care, regardless of geographical or economic barriers.

With these technologies at our fingertips, the field of animal behavior analysis is set for profound change. AI doesn't just offer new solutions; it reshapes the fundamental questions we've long asked about animal care and behavior. As we embrace these tools, our connection with animals strengthens, fueled by a deeper understanding of their needs and experiences. And in turn, we are inspired to create a world where animals, both domestic and wild, can live with dignity and joy.

Chapter 12:
Ethics and AI in Veterinary Medicine

As AI transforms veterinary medicine, the ethical implications can't be overlooked. Balancing the promise of innovation with the responsible use of technology is crucial for maintaining trust and ensuring animal welfare. With AI-driven diagnostics and treatment plans becoming more prevalent, veterinarians face new moral dilemmas. There's a pressing need to establish guidelines for the responsible development and deployment of AI, ensuring these systems enhance, rather than hinder, the quality of care. Striking a balance between technological advancement and compassionate animal care requires ongoing dialogue among stakeholders, ranging from practitioners to tech developers. By approaching these challenges with a commitment to transparency and ethical rigor, the veterinary community can harness AI's potential while safeguarding the foundational values of veterinary practice.

Responsible AI Use

The integration of artificial intelligence in veterinary medicine opens promising avenues for enhancing healthcare, improving diagnostics, and personalizing treatments for animals. However, alongside these opportunities comes the responsibility of ensuring AI's ethical use. Veterinarians, technologists, and animal caregivers must work together to embrace AI innovations responsibly, ensuring that benefits are maximized and risks are minimized. This chapter aims to address the necessity for responsible AI use as it reshapes veterinary practices, advocating for ethical guidelines and frameworks.

One of the foremost considerations is ensuring that AI development prioritizes animal welfare above all else. It's crucial that AI systems do not merely replace human judgment but augment it, facilitating a deeper understanding and care for animal health. This requires transparency from developers regarding how AI systems are trained and tested. Clear documentation should be in place to ensure that these systems align with ethical veterinary practices.

Data privacy is another cornerstone of responsible AI use. The massive amount of data collected and processed by AI systems includes sensitive information about animals and their owners. Safeguarding this data is imperative to prevent breaches that could compromise privacy and trust. Veterinarians should be informed and vigilant about the security measures employed by AI technologies they adopt, ensuring compliance with privacy regulations and ethical standards.

Bias in AI algorithms is a significant concern that must be addressed. If algorithms are trained on datasets that lack diversity or are unrepresentative of the broader animal population, it can lead to biased outcomes. This can result in inaccurate diagnoses or inappropriate treatment recommendations. Continuous efforts are needed to identify and eliminate biases, requiring collaboration between data scientists, veterinarians, and ethicists to develop inclusive and equitable AI models.

Another aspect of responsible AI use involves ensuring that the adoption of AI doesn't lead to the deskilling of veterinary professionals. AI should be viewed as a tool that enhances human capabilities, providing insights and efficiencies that were previously unattainable. Education and training programs play a vital role in equipping veterinarians with skills to effectively collaborate with AI technologies, thus enriching their professional expertise rather than diminishing it.

The environmental impact of AI technologies cannot be overlooked. The computational power required to develop and run sophisticated AI systems often demands significant energy resources. Promoting sustainability in AI development is essential, encouraging practices that minimize environmental footprints. Veterinarians and AI developers should advocate for greener technologies and consider the ecological ramifications of AI applications in veterinary medicine.

Furthermore, the ethical implications of AI's decision-making abilities must be scrutinized. While AI can process vast datasets and recognize patterns beyond human capacity, it lacks the ability to comprehend the emotional and situational nuances unique to living creatures. Decisions affecting animal treatment and care should always involve human oversight, ensuring that moral and ethical considerations remain central to veterinary practice.

Collaboration between the veterinary community, AI developers, and regulatory bodies is essential to establishing and upholding standards for responsible AI use. A proactive approach involves veterinarians voicing their needs and challenges, allowing developers to tailor AI solutions that are both ethical and practical. Regulatory bodies should continuously update guidelines to reflect advances in AI, ensuring they are relevant and effective in protecting animal welfare.

The continuous monitoring and evaluation of AI systems in practice should be prioritized, creating feedback loops that ensure AI tools adapt and evolve responsibly. Commitment from all stakeholders to engage in ongoing dialogue ensures that AI continues to benefit animal and human health while adhering to ethical standards. Such vigilance helps to build trust in AI technologies and reinforces their positive role in veterinary medicine.

Finally, as AI becomes increasingly embedded in veterinary care, it's essential to cultivate a community that champions responsible AI use. This involves not only adhering to guidelines and best practices but also fostering a culture that values ethical considerations as much as technological advancements. Animal welfare should remain at the forefront, guiding every decision and innovation in AI veterinary applications.

In conclusion, the responsible use of AI in veterinary medicine hinges on carefully balancing innovation with ethical oversight. It requires a collective effort from veterinarians, developers, policymakers, and the broader society to realize AI's full potential in enhancing animal health care. As we move forward, our commitment to responsible AI use will ultimately shape the future of veterinary medicine, ensuring it serves both animals and humans with integrity and compassion.

Balancing Innovation with Care

As artificial intelligence continues to make waves in the world of veterinary medicine, the excitement surrounding its potential is palpable. AI promises to revolutionize diagnostics, treatment plans, and animal care, offering unprecedented insights and efficiencies. But amidst this whirlwind of technological advancement, one must pause and consider the ethical implications of integrating AI into veterinary practice. Balancing innovation with care becomes a delicate dance, one that requires vigilance, thoughtful consideration, and a deep understanding of the responsibilities we hold toward our animal companions.

It's crucial to recognize that the primary goal of veterinary medicine has always been to promote the health and well-being of animals. This goal shouldn't waver as we introduce AI into the equation. AI can offer rapid data analysis and predictive accuracy, which are incredibly beneficial in clinical settings. However, the emphasis must remain on using these tools to enhance, not replace, the empathetic care practiced by veterinarians. Putting animal welfare at the forefront ensures that technology serves as a bridge and not a barrier to compassionate care.

One of the fundamental ethical challenges is ensuring that AI tools are unbiased and equitable. Algorithms, after all, are trained on data, and if this data isn't representative of diverse animal populations, it can lead to skewed results. Imagine an AI tool designed for diagnostic imaging that's primarily trained on data from certain breeds but falls short when analyzing another. This discrepancy isn't just a technical issue—it's an ethical one, highlighting the importance of diverse data sets and continuous algorithmic updates.

Veterinarians are no strangers to the complexity of ethical decision-making. They've always walked the fine line between offering the best care possible and considering the economic constraints of their clients. As AI enters the scene, it introduces new layers to these decisions. AI tools can offer recommendations based on vast datasets and clinical history, but the final decisions should always involve the expertise and intuition of trained professionals. The human element in veterinary medicine remains irreplaceable, ensuring that AI augments rather than dictates the course of treatment.

Another aspect of balancing innovation with care lies in the integration of AI tools in ways that do not overwhelm caregivers or disrupt existing workflows. Veterinarians must be given proper training to use these technologies effectively and responsibly. Implementing AI solutions should never become a burden that detracts from the time and attention that animals need. Instead, it should be a process that respects and possibly enhances the caregivers' ability to deliver personalized and compassionate care.

Transparency with pet owners is also paramount. As clients begin to encounter AI-driven recommendations in veterinary settings, they will naturally have questions and concerns. Open communication about how these tools work and the data they use can foster trust between veterinarians and pet owners. Transparency ensures clients feel confident in the new technologies complementing traditional care, rather than viewing them as foreign or unreliable.

Privacy is yet another area requiring attentive consideration. AI systems often rely on vast amounts of data to improve and learn. Ensuring that this data is securely handled and that client confidentiality is maintained is crucial. Policies around data collection and usage must be clearly communicated to pet owners to mitigate any potential mistrust or misunderstandings. The veterinary sector must forge paths that honor privacy while reaping the benefits of shared knowledge across the industry.

Looking forward, balancing innovation with care also means being proactive about potential ethical dilemmas. The rapid pace of technological advances can sometimes outstrip our ability to address associated moral questions. To counteract this, those working at the intersection of AI and veterinary medicine must engage in continuous dialogue, examining emerging technologies from ethical standpoints and anticipating issues before they arise. It's an ongoing conversation that requires input from veterinarians, AI experts, ethicists, and even the public. This collective vigilance ensures that innovation in veterinary AI doesn't just advance knowledge and capabilities but does so conscientiously and humanely.

It's easy to get swept up in the promise of AI—a field moving with dizzying speed and offering solutions once thought impossible. But in this technological renaissance, we must keep our foundational values in sight. Technology should empower veterinarians, enabling them to spend more time understanding and addressing the nuances of each animal's needs. Only by holding fast to the principles of thoughtful and ethical integration can AI truly become a tool that enriches the lives of animals and the humans who care for them.

Ultimately, the future of veterinary medicine with AI looks bright, but it's up to us to steer it responsibly. Fostering a careful equilibrium between innovation and care ensures that as AI technologies evolve, they enhance the profession and, most importantly, the lives of the animals we cherish. So, while we harness the power of AI, let's do so with consideration, ensuring that every leap forward is a step toward more compassionate and effective veterinary care.

Chapter 13:
AI in Veterinary Education

As the landscape of veterinary medicine evolves with the integration of artificial intelligence, the education of aspiring veterinarians is undergoing a transformative shift. AI is not just a tool for the practice; it's becoming an essential part of the curriculum, preparing students for a future where technology and healing converge. Through AI-enhanced learning tools, such as virtual reality simulations and interactive models, students gain hands-on experience with complex procedures in a risk-free environment. This innovative approach allows them to master diagnostic techniques and surgical skills with unprecedented precision. Moreover, AI aids in tailoring educational experiences to individual learning styles, ensuring that each student can grasp intricate concepts effectively. The next generation of veterinarians will enter the field not only with traditional knowledge but also with a robust understanding of AI applications, ready to harness these cutting-edge technologies in delivering advanced animal care.

Training the Next Generation

As artificial intelligence (AI) continues to revolutionize veterinary medicine, the focus shifts toward an equally important frontier: education. Training the next generation of veterinarians not only involves imparting traditional medical knowledge but also understanding and integrating cutting-edge AI technologies. This new era of veterinary education promises to better equip practitioners to handle the complexities of modern animal healthcare.

The foundation of incorporating AI into veterinary education lies in understanding the synergy between technology and clinical acumen. Future veterinarians are expected to harness AI tools effectively, which requires a curriculum that balances classical veterinary education with robust technological training. By introducing courses that delve into machine learning, data analytics, and AI ethics, veterinary schools can prepare students to leverage AI in practice while maintaining a strong ethical compass.

A transformative approach in this educational journey is the inclusion of practical, AI-driven learning experiences. Virtual simulations and interactive modules powered by AI allow students to engage with realistic clinical scenarios. This hands-on experience helps them to not only learn diagnostics and decision-making in a risk-free environment but also to appreciate the nuanced interpretations AI can offer. As a result, students can cultivate adaptable skill sets, giving them the agility to address diverse veterinary challenges.

Integrating AI into veterinary education also encourages collaboration across disciplines. Veterinary students are exposed to interdisciplinary knowledge, collaborating with AI experts, computer scientists, and data analysts. Such collaborative learning fosters an environment where students understand the multifaceted nature of AI. By bridging the gap between disciplines, educators can cultivate an ecosystem of innovation where students are encouraged to explore AI's potential in animal healthcare.

Mentorship plays an equally significant role in this transformation. Leading veterinarians who are well-versed in AI applications serve as mentors, guiding students through the intricacies of AI-enabled veterinary care. Their expertise provides invaluable insights into the real-world implementation of AI, highlighting both its advantages and limitations. Mentorship thus ensures that the next generation of veterinarians is competent in critical thinking and confident in using AI tools, preparing them to pioneer new solutions in animal health.

Additionally, the integration of AI in veterinary education calls for the continuous evolution of teaching methodologies. Adaptive learning platforms that employ AI to tailor educational content based on an individual student's learning pattern are gaining traction. Such platforms facilitate personalized learning experiences, ensuring that each student can progress at their own pace while mastering the curriculum. Through AI-enhanced learning tools, students are encouraged to develop their strengths while strategically addressing their weaknesses.

However, the integration of AI into education isn't without challenges. There are concerns about the accessibility of such advanced technologies. Educational institutions must strive to provide equal opportunities by ensuring that all students, regardless of background, have access to AI learning tools. This may include partnerships with technology companies to secure resources and funding or developing open-source platforms that democratize access to AI methodologies.

Moreover, educators must balance the technological aspects with the humanistic elements of veterinary practice. AI should enhance human capabilities, not overshadow them. Emphasizing the compassionate and emotional aspects of veterinary care ensures that future veterinarians remain empathetic caregivers, despite the increasing prevalence of technology. By cultivating emotional intelligence alongside technical expertise, veterinary education can prepare practitioners who are both skilled and compassionate.

As veterinary medicine evolves with AI, it's crucial to instill a sense of ethical responsibility in students. This involves fostering an understanding of the socio-ethical implications of AI in medicine. Curriculums should engage students in discussions about data privacy, the potential for bias in AI algorithms, and the equitable use of AI technologies. Educators can inspire students to champion ethical AI practices, ensuring that this powerful technology is used responsibly and inclusively.

In conclusion, training the next generation of veterinarians in the age of AI requires a comprehensive educational approach. By blending traditional veterinary knowledge with AI-focused courses, providing hands-on AI experiences, fostering interdisciplinary collaboration, and maintaining ethical standards, veterinary schools can prepare students to lead in the future of animal healthcare. As these future veterinarians enter the workforce, they'll be equipped not only with the skills to utilize AI effectively but also with the vision to innovate and transform veterinary medicine, ensuring the well-being of animals across the globe.

AI-Enhanced Learning Tools

In an era where technology shapes nearly every facet of our lives, veterinary education is on the brink of a transformative evolution with AI-enhanced learning tools at the forefront. These tools are not just changing how veterinary students absorb information but also how they interact with their future workplace environments. Imagine a classroom where each student can explore a holographic model of a canine heart, rotate it, dissect it virtually, and see the effects of various diseases in real-time. This is no longer science fiction but a burgeoning reality, reshaping the learning landscape.

AI-enhanced tools in veterinary education blend theoretical knowledge with practical implementation, providing students with immersive, interactive experiences. This approach helps bridge the gap between textbook-learning and hands-on veterinary practice. Tools such as virtual reality (VR) and augmented reality (AR) are finding their way into lecture halls, simulating complex surgical procedures or replicating animal behaviors for analysis. These technologies allow students to repeatedly practice techniques, thereby reinforcing learning and building confidence before they ever enter a real veterinary clinic. The ability to "learn by doing" in a risk-free environment is a significant leap forward.

Machine learning algorithms are becoming indispensable tutors in the realm of veterinary education. They personalize learning experiences by adapting to the pace and style of individual students, ensuring no one is left behind. For instance, AI can assess a student's understanding and offer custom-tailored quizzes and feedback. This adaptive learning technology fosters autonomy, accountability, and self-directed growth, vital qualities in any proficient veterinarian. With every interaction, these systems gather data to refine their teaching methods, ultimately empowering educators to focus on more complex instructional challenges.

Real-world case studies form another integral component of AI-enhanced learning. By integrating big data, AI systems can present students with dynamic, ever-evolving clinical scenarios. These scenarios can reflect the latest veterinary research or rare cases sourced globally, providing a context-rich learning experience that textbooks alone can't offer. As students navigate these realistic cases, they learn to apply their diagnostic skills efficiently, honing their critical thinking and decision-making abilities.

Content delivery isn't limited to the four walls of a classroom. Distance learning has gained momentum, and AI plays a pivotal role in expanding the reach of veterinary education beyond geographical boundaries. Through e-learning platforms, students can engage with interactive modules from anywhere in the world, receiving instantaneous feedback from AI-driven assessments. This accessibility democratizes education, allowing aspiring veterinarians from underserved regions to participate in world-class training without the need for physical relocation, thereby broadening the diversity and inclusivity of the veterinary profession.

Equally transformative is the role of AI in facilitating collaborative learning environments. Modern veterinary education thrives on interdisciplinary collaboration, and AI tools support this by enabling seamless communication and idea sharing among students from diverse backgrounds. Virtual classrooms and AI-enabled discussion forums foster a sense of community, where knowledge is built collectively. This collaborative spirit is crucial for fostering innovative problem-solving skills, essential for tackling the multifaceted challenges that veterinary medicine presents.

Furthermore, AI-enhanced learning tools are gradually incorporating elements of gamification to boost engagement and motivation. By introducing game-like elements into educational content, such as point scoring, leaderboards, or badges for achievements, students are more likely to remain engaged and retain information better. Learning becomes an exciting journey rather than a monotonous obligation, encouraging consistent participation and deeper understanding.

Despite the myriad benefits AI-enhanced learning brings, it's essential to acknowledge and address potential challenges. Privacy concerns, data security, and ensuring unbiased algorithms are paramount considerations. As these technologies gather and analyze a vast range of student data, maintaining ethical standards in handling and utilizing this information is crucial. Moreover, educators must be equipped to integrate these technologies effectively into existing curriculums, which requires continuous training and upskilling.

The potential of AI to shape the future of veterinary education is immense, and the journey is just beginning. As tools continue to evolve, they offer unprecedented opportunities to transform both the teaching and practice of veterinary medicine. As learners today harness these technologies, they are better prepared to respond to the complex and dynamic challenges of tomorrow's veterinary landscape, ensuring that the next generation of veterinarians is more skilled, knowledgeable, and adaptable than ever before. The integration of AI in education is not merely a technological upgrade; it is a paradigm shift toward a more interactive, personalized, and comprehensive learning experience.

Chapter 14:
AI and Emergency Veterinary Care

AI is revolutionizing emergency veterinary care, pushing the boundaries of what's possible during those critical, life-or-death moments. In the chaos of an emergency, rapid decision-making is paramount, and AI technologies are stepping in as vital allies. With sophisticated algorithms, veterinarians can prioritize patients quickly, efficiently identifying those in dire need through AI-driven triage systems. These systems analyze data from wearable devices and medical history at lightning speed, assisting vets in making informed decisions when every second counts. During crisis situations, AI tools provide real-time insights and predictive analytics that support swift interventions, ensuring timely care and improving survival rates. As machines learn from countless emergency scenarios, they're constantly refining their ability to assist with split-second judgments, effectively transforming chaotic moments into coordinated responses. This blend of human expertise and AI prowess is setting new standards in emergency veterinary care, offering hope when it's needed most.

Rapid Triage and Decision-Making

In the throes of an emergency, every moment counts, and having the capability to make rapid, informed decisions can be the difference between life and death for a beloved animal. AI-powered tools are transforming the landscape of emergency veterinary care, providing unparalleled speed and efficiency in assessing critical situations.

At the heart of this transformation is the ability of AI systems to rapidly collect and analyze vast amounts of data. These systems can bring together information from the animal's medical history, real-time monitoring, and diagnostic tools to quickly assess the situation. This integrated approach enables veterinarians to triage cases with a level of precision that was previously unattainable.

A key advantage of AI in this arena is its capability to process complex data sets in real-time. For example, when an animal is rushed in with symptoms of a heart condition, AI can immediately analyze ECG patterns, compare them with millions of other cases, and suggest potential diagnoses. This rapid analysis supports the veterinarian's clinical judgment, helping them to prioritize interventions and focus their efforts on the most critical aspects of care.

AI doesn't just assist with speed but also with complexity. Emergency cases often involve a myriad of variables, and AI tools are particularly adept at making sense of these multifaceted situations. For instance, in cases of poisoning, the AI can cross-reference the symptoms, possible toxic agents, and suggested treatments with existing databases to streamline decision-making processes. This approach reduces the guesswork and helps mitigate the risks inherent in emergency treatment.

Moreover, AI systems are learning continuously, improving their understanding of numerous emergency conditions every time they are used. This iterative learning means that AI tools are not static; they constantly adapt and refine their suggestions, making them increasingly valuable resources over time. As more veterinary professionals adopt such technologies, the collective knowledge base grows, potentially leading to even more effective emergency responses.

Yet, the incorporation of AI into emergency veterinary care is not just about speed and accuracy; it also supports emotional decision-making burdens. Managing an emergency situation can be a highly stressful experience for veterinarians, who must often make swift decisions under pressure. AI provides an objective layer of support that can help professionals feel more confident in their choices, allowing them to manage stress better and focus on delivering compassionate care.

Consider the implications of a tool that allows quick triage during mass casualty events in wildlife, such as oil spills or natural disasters. AI systems can assist veterinarians by identifying and grouping the most critical cases, ensuring that the limited resources available are directed where they're needed most. The ability to prioritize effectively can drastically improve outcomes in what are otherwise overwhelming scenarios.

Additionally, AI is enhancing communication within the veterinary team and with pet owners. Decision-making processes become transparent and data-driven, which helps build trust and understanding. Pet owners are likely to feel more reassured when they see that their animal's care involves cutting-edge technology and thorough data analysis, which can reduce anxiety in emergency situations.

One should also appreciate the potential integration of AI into telemedicine platforms, which can offer remote triage services. In areas where immediate access to a veterinary hospital isn't possible, AI tools can guide pet owners and suggest initial care measures while they prepare to transport their pet. This capability can significantly enhance outcomes by ensuring early intervention.

Nevertheless, the implementation of AI in emergency care isn't without challenges. It's crucial to remember that AI serves as a supportive tool rather than a replacement for human expertise. The ultimate decision-making power still rests with the veterinarians who must interpret AI recommendations within the broader context of each unique case.

An essential aspect of this integration is also the ethical considerations it entails. As AI takes on more significant roles in decision-making, defining the boundaries and responsibilities becomes critical. How accountable should an AI system be for a recommendation that doesn't lead to a favorable outcome? This question is vital in shaping the future of AI in emergency care.

Training and familiarization with AI systems are of paramount importance. Veterinary teams need adequate training to harness these tools effectively. This training ensures that AI solutions are used to their fullest potential, promoting both rapid response and accurate decision-making during emergencies.

In conclusion, the advent of AI in rapid triage and decision-making is a pivotal development in the field of emergency veterinary care. By enhancing data analysis, providing insightful recommendations, and supporting veterinary teams in their critical work, AI is paving the way for an evolution in how emergencies are managed. By bridging technology with empathy, AI not only empowers veterinarians but also ensures animals receive the utmost care when they need it most.

AI in Crisis Situations

In the fast-paced world of veterinary medicine, crises demand rapid, informed decision-making. Recently, the incorporation of artificial intelligence (AI) has transformed the way veterinarians handle emergencies, providing them not just with tools to manage these situations but also offering a safety net that was once unimaginable. From natural disasters affecting large populations of animals to individual pets experiencing sudden medical emergencies, AI's role in orchestrating efficient crisis management is revolutionary.

One of the primary strengths of AI in crisis situations lies in its ability to rapidly triage cases. AI systems can swiftly analyze symptoms, compare them against a vast database of historical cases, and prioritize treatment for animals most in need of immediate attention. This process, once reliant on the human capacity to quickly assess and make educated guesses under pressure, is now supported by intelligent algorithms that increase accuracy and decrease the time spent in decision-making.

Imagine a scenario where a sudden outbreak of disease spreads through a wildlife sanctuary. The logistics of traditional methods, involving lengthy data analysis followed by ground-level response coordination, could prove detrimental. Here, AI enables real-time surveillance and data collation, providing vital insights into disease progression and transmission patterns. AI's analytical prowess doesn't just inform veterinary teams but also empowers them with actionable data, facilitating quicker response times and more effective containment strategies.

Crisis intervention benefits immensely from AI-driven predictive analytics. Equipped with machine learning models trained on vast datasets, these systems can forecast the trajectory of health emergencies before they peak. For example, during an epidemic threatening a community of livestock, AI can predict potential outbreaks through subtle changes in data, such as environmental factors, animal behavior, and even emerging patterns not immediately visible to the human eye.

During disasters, communication and coordination become pivotal. AI helps streamline these processes, providing a unified interface that connects disparate teams and systems. A centralized AI platform ensures that all stakeholders—from veterinarians and field agents to support staff and decision-makers—have access to the same, real-time information. This interconnectedness reduces redundancies and enhances the efficiency of crisis response operations.

Equally important is AI's role in educating and preparing veterinary teams for emergencies. By simulating various crisis scenarios,

AI can help train personnel, enabling them to rehearse responses to a myriad of emergencies in a controlled, virtual environment. This preparation not only increases the competence of individual practitioners but also fosters cohesive team dynamics when real-life crises emerge, where every second counts.

AI's ability to assist in decision-making during emergencies is bolstered by its capacity to operate independently in certain scenarios. For emergencies that demand immediate attention—such as an animal suffering from acute distress in a remote location—autonomous AI systems can provide immediate intervention. These systems can stabilize the patient using automated medical tools, offering supportive care until human help can arrive.

The utility of AI in crisis situations isn't confined to just medical interventions. During large-scale emergencies, such as natural disasters, AI plays a crucial role in logistical support, ensuring that necessary supplies, equipment, and personnel are routed to where they are most needed, effectively optimizing resource deployment and minimizing response times.

However, the implementation of AI in crisis situations also requires ethical considerations. The adoption of AI technologies must be carefully balanced with empathy and human oversight to ensure decisions align with humane treatment principles. While AI can assist in making assessments, it is ultimately up to veterinary professionals to contextualize this information and make the final decisions, ensuring the primary focus remains on compassionate care.

As AI continues to evolve, its potential applications in crisis management are vast and varied. Advanced AI systems are on the horizon, capable of learning from each crisis to improve their response mechanisms and predictive accuracy. These systems, evolving through machine learning and other AI technologies, promise a future where veterinary aid in emergencies is even more reliable and efficient than it is today.

Furthermore, AI has the potential to democratize emergency care by providing access to tools and insights to veterinarians in remote or underserved areas. This broadens the reach of quality care, ensuring that no community or animal population is left unsupported during times of crisis. Equipping veterinary teams worldwide with AI-driven capabilities will undoubtedly lead to a more resilient global response network for animal health crises.

In conclusion, AI is steadily becoming an invaluable ally in the field of emergency veterinary care. Its ability to assist in rapid decision-making, optimize resource allocation, and support crisis management through real-time data analysis and autonomous functions heralds a new era of veterinary medicine. As veterinarians embrace these innovations, AI's integration promises not only to transform individual emergency responses but also to redefine the landscape of animal healthcare during critical situations.

Chapter 15:
AI for Large Animal and Livestock Care

In the evolving landscape of veterinary medicine, AI is revolutionizing the care and management of large animals and livestock, bringing smart, data-driven solutions to age-old agricultural challenges. This chapter delves into how artificial intelligence is optimizing farm management and enhancing livestock health, offering a glimpse into a future where efficiency and sustainability go hand-in-hand. Through predictive analytics, farmers can foresee health issues before they manifest, turning potential crises into manageable events. AI tools analyze weather patterns, optimize feeding schedules, and ensure precise herd management, minimizing wastage while maximizing productivity. Furthermore, comprehensive health monitoring systems provide veterinarians with real-time data, enabling precise interventions that improve overall animal well-being. Such innovations not only bolster the efficiency of livestock operations but also ensure ethical standards and animal welfare are upheld. As we navigate through these technological advances, AI emerges as a pivotal ally in crafting a new era of integrated, smart agricultural practices.

Optimizing Farm Management

As agricultural practices face mounting pressures from climate change, population growth, and resource scarcity, the necessity for innovative solutions has never been greater. AI-driven technologies offer remarkable opportunities to revolutionize farm management, particularly in large animal and livestock care. By harnessing the power of artificial intelligence, farmers can streamline operations, enhance productivity, and promote sustainable practices.

To optimize farm management, AI systems can integrate data from various sources such as weather forecasts, soil sensors, and market trends. This fusion of data provides farmers with real-time insights into crop conditions and potential challenges. While the past relied heavily on manual labor and intuition, today's farms can leverage sophisticated algorithms to predict the best times for planting, harvesting, and rotating crops. These algorithms consider numerous variables: soil moisture levels, nutrient availability, and weather patterns, making recommendations that align with optimal growth conditions.

Livestock management is benefiting immensely from AI technologies, primarily through the automation of daily tasks. Feeding, watering, and health monitoring can all be controlled via smart systems, reducing the potential for human error and ensuring animals are cared for consistently. The labor-intensive chores that once dominated a farmer's day are now streamlined, allowing more time to be focused on higher-level decision-making and strategic planning.

Moreover, AI tools help analyze animal behavior to optimize welfare and productivity. By using computer vision and machine learning, farmers can track movement patterns and identify signs of distress or illness long before they manifest physically. This proactive approach enables early intervention, reducing the risk of severe outbreaks and improving overall herd health. Not only does this foster a better quality of life for the animals, but it also contributes to higher yields and economic gains.

In terms of resource management, AI systems can significantly reduce waste and improve sustainability. Sensors that monitor feed intake and conversion rates allow farmers to adjust nutrition regimens, ensuring livestock receive precisely what they need without excess. This precision feeding, guided by AI, minimizes costs and enhances growth rates, reducing the environmental impact of livestock farming through lower emissions and better use of natural resources.

AI also plays a critical role in economic optimization by analyzing market trends and demand forecasting. Predictive analytics allow farmers to make informed decisions about when to sell their products, maximizing profits while minimizing risk during market fluctuations. These insights ensure that farms remain viable even when external economic pressures, such as price volatility or trade disruptions, arise.

Simultaneously, the transition towards AI-integrated farm management isn't without its challenges. Farmers face barriers such as the initial costs of technology adoption, the need for ongoing training, and the balancing act between technological and traditional practices. Yet by partnering with tech companies and engaging with initiatives that provide funding or subsidies, these obstacles can be gradually overcome. As the adoption of AI continues to spread throughout the industry, its benefits become increasingly accessible to farms of all sizes.

The shift to AI couldn't come at a more pivotal time. As the agricultural industry strives for sustainable practices, setting its sights on long-term viability, AI provides the tools needed for this transformation. It empowers farmers not merely as stewards of the land but as pioneers of innovation. These tools create an ecosystem where efficiency meets empathy, allowing for the care of animals and the planet to be achieved harmoniously.

Though AI in agriculture is still in its formative years, its potential is boundless. From small, family-owned operations to expansive commercial enterprises, the scalable nature of these technologies means no farm is too small or too large to benefit. As AI continues to evolve, integrating more seamless and intelligent systems will redefine what's possible in farm management, marking a thrilling frontier in agriculture.

Without a doubt, the incorporation of AI into farm management signifies more than a technological advancement—it's a paradigm shift. The opportunity to enhance productivity while reducing ecological footprints creates a promising outlook for both farmers and consumers. In shaping this future, AI stands not just as a tool but as a partner in nurturing an agricultural landscape that prioritizes health and prosperity for generations to come.

Enhancing Livestock Health

The intersection of AI and livestock health promises to revolutionize the agricultural industry. Livestock health is critical not only for animal welfare but also for the economic stability of farmers and the global food supply chain. Maintaining the health of every animal on a farm is a herculean task, and this is where AI steps in as a game-changer. AI technologies allow farmers to identify illness before it spreads, administer precise treatments, and improve the overall care of livestock.

Automation and data collection offer significant breakthroughs. Farmers can use AI-powered cameras and sensors to continually monitor livestock. These devices track everything from body temperature and movement patterns to feed and water intake. Such constant surveillance was once only possible with human oversight, often impractical on large farms. AI streamlines this process by instantly flagging abnormalities that could signify health issues long before they become visible to the naked eye.

Moreover, AI enhances diagnostic capabilities. Traditional methods of identifying diseases can be labor-intensive and time-consuming. AI can speed up this process, analyzing vast amounts of data more quickly and accurately than humans. By using machine learning algorithms, AI can identify subtle patterns in health data that might indicate the onset of disease. This level of precision ensures that interventions can happen earlier, reducing mortality rates and increasing the productivity of livestock.

Imagine a world where a farmer receives an alert on their smartphone notifying them that a cow in the back pasture shows signs of distress. AI makes it possible by integrating with smart devices, providing timely alerts and recommendations. This connectivity allows for quick assessments and interventions that were previously unmanageable. With detailed reports at their fingertips, farmers can prioritize animal welfare, ultimately leading to healthier herds and improved yield.

In addition to detection, AI plays a pivotal role in treatment. It offers tailored solutions based on individual animal needs. By leveraging predictive analytics, AI can recommend customized treatment plans, ensuring livestock receive the right medicine in the right dosages. Such precision minimizes waste and reduces the potential for antibiotic resistance, a growing concern in animal care.

Furthermore, automated systems can administer these treatments efficiently and consistently. Farmers, who traditionally might struggle with administering the correct dosages, especially across large herds, now have AI-driven systems that can apply medicine with pinpoint accuracy. This automation not only saves time but also improves the effectiveness of treatments, leading to faster recovery times and healthier animals.

AI's influence extends beyond individual animal care to herd management strategies. Through predictive analytics, AI helps farmers make informed decisions regarding breeding and herd dynamics. It examines a combination of health data, environmental conditions, and historical trends to suggest optimal breeding cycles and herd compositions. Such strategies contribute to healthier, more resilient livestock populations, capable of withstanding the challenges posed by climate change and evolving global demands.

Feed optimization is another area where AI excels. Livestock nutrition plays a significant role in health outcomes, yet managing dietary needs across different animals can be complex. AI-driven platforms analyze data from various sources, such as nutrition requirements, health records, and growth patterns, to suggest diets tailored to specific needs. By ensuring that each animal receives precisely what it needs, AI contributes to improved growth rates and overall herd vitality.

The integration of AI in livestock health also holds promise in addressing zoonotic diseases. Zoonoses, diseases transmissible from animals to humans, pose significant risks to public health. With AI's ability to identify early warning signs and track disease spread, it becomes a crucial tool in preventing outbreaks. By using AI to predict and quarantine affected animals, we can significantly reduce the risks associated with these diseases.

There's also an environmental dimension to consider. Sustainable livestock management is a pressing concern as the agriculture industry grapples with its environmental footprint. AI helps optimize resource use by accurately predicting the needs of livestock, lowering the reliance on water and feed. This efficiency reduces waste and lessens the environmental impact of farming operations, contributing to a more sustainable future.

Indeed, for many, AI still raises concerns about its complexity and the learning curve associated with new technologies. However, the rise of AI in livestock health emphasizes its accessibility and effectiveness rather than its difficulty. Solutions are increasingly user-friendly, with interfaces designed with farmers in mind. Education and integration could empower more in the agricultural community to embrace these transformative tools, easing transitions and maximizing benefits.

The social and economic implications of enhancing livestock health with AI are profound. As farming operations become more efficient and productive, they can achieve higher yields and decrease losses, supporting local economies and pushing agriculture forward worldwide. Enhanced livestock health also means improved food quality, meeting consumer demands for safe and nutritious products.

Ultimately, the implementation of AI in livestock health signifies a transformation in veterinary care practices. It embodies an opportunity for humanity to reframe how we approach animal well-being, recognizing our interdependence and working towards a future that promotes the health of all species. With AI's promise, livestock health can become not just about maintaining the status quo but striving for an unprecedented standard of excellence and care. As we look towards the future, the prospects of AI in livestock health are not merely enhancements but a pivotal shift towards sustainable and humane farming practices.

Chapter 16:
AI in Veterinary Genomics

The fusion of artificial intelligence and veterinary genomics is creating new pathways for understanding and enhancing animal health. By leveraging AI algorithms capable of analyzing vast amounts of genetic data, veterinarians are unlocking insights into the genetic makeup of various species. These insights empower precise genetic testing and analysis, revealing predispositions to diseases and unlocking opportunities for tailored health interventions. AI plays a pivotal role in guiding informed breeding decisions, aiming for traits that optimize health and vitality. This revolution in genomics allows for proactive disease prevention strategies and promotes a future where veterinary care is more predictive and personalized. As we harness the potential of AI, it not only illuminates the path to healthier animals but also fortifies biodiversity by preserving genome integrity across generations.

Genetic Testing and Analysis

The integration of artificial intelligence into veterinary genomics is opening new horizons for genetic testing and analysis, transforming how veterinary professionals approach animal healthcare. By harnessing AI, veterinarians can decipher complex genetic information rapidly and with greater accuracy, tailoring healthcare strategies to the unique genetic makeup of each animal. This capacity to analyze and interpret genomic data efficiently is ushering in a new era of personalized veterinary medicine.

At the heart of this transformation is the ability of AI to handle vast amounts of genetic data. Genomic sequencing generates enormous datasets, often too large and complicated for traditional analysis approaches. AI algorithms, particularly those utilizing machine learning, can sift through these data troves swiftly. They not only identify known genetic variants but also predict potential unknown mutations that might affect an animal's health. By understanding these genetic markers, veterinarians can diagnose hereditary diseases at a much earlier stage, greatly improving treatment outcomes.

AI's role doesn't stop at disease diagnosis. It plays a crucial part in developing comprehensive genetic profiles for animals, which can guide breeding programs to enhance the health and vitality of future generations. This is particularly relevant in breeding animals for particular traits, but with a responsible approach, focusing on health-related traits rather than just aesthetic ones. AI can help ensure genetic diversity, reducing the risk of health issues associated with inbreeding by analyzing genetic similarities and variances across populations.

The precision that AI brings to genetic testing extends further into predicting disease susceptibility. For instance, through predictive modeling, AI can evaluate an animal's risk for developing certain conditions based on their genotype. This proactive approach allows veterinarians and pet owners to implement preventive measures much earlier. Moreover, insights gained can assist in drawing family histories in animals more accurately, giving breeders and owners critical tools to make informed decisions about animal care and management.

Moreover, AI is refining the methodology of genomic editing. Techniques like CRISPR for gene editing are being augmented with AI to improve accuracy and efficiency. AI-driven models can predict how changes to an animal's genome might manifest, minimizing risks and ensuring that only beneficial changes are made. This ensures healthier lineages and can potentially eradicate hereditary conditions from animal populations.

The benefits of AI in genetic testing and analysis extend to wildlife conservation efforts as well. By analyzing genetic data from wildlife populations, conservationists can identify genetic markers that indicate vulnerability to specific diseases or environmental changes. AI can also track genetic diversity within and between populations, aiding in the development of conservation strategies that augment genetic resilience and sustain biodiversity.

For veterinary professionals, these advancements mean a shift in skill requirements. Veterinary genomic analysis now demands proficiency in AI technologies, as understanding the output from AI-driven genomic tools is crucial for accurate interpretation and application. Continuous education will be essential as the technology evolves, ensuring veterinarians remain at the forefront of genetic science.

While AI-powered genetic testing and analysis promise numerous benefits, ethical considerations cannot be overlooked. The potential for genetic manipulation requires careful regulation to prevent misuse, and privacy concerns surrounding genetic data must be addressed. Developing comprehensive, ethical guidelines for AI use in this context is essential to ensure that technology serves the best interest of animal welfare.

AI is undoubtedly revolutionizing genetic testing and analysis in veterinary genomics, making it possible to offer more personalized, effective, and ethical care. This technological innovation empowers veterinarians to take proactive measures, improving diagnoses and treatment and offering the potential to fundamentally alter the landscape of animal health management. As AI continues to evolve, it will undeniably lead to even more groundbreaking developments in veterinary genomics.

Breeding for Improved Health

In the ever-evolving landscape of veterinary genomics, artificial intelligence is charting pathways that once seemed the realm of science fiction. The synergy between AI and genomics is reshaping traditional breeding methods, offering unprecedented insights into genetic markers that influence animal health. For veterinarians and tech enthusiasts alike, this is an exciting frontier where science meets compassion, aiming to engineer healthier, more resilient animals.

Traditional breeding has always been a mixture of art and science, with breeders selecting animals based on visible traits and informed speculation about their genetic makeup. However, AI is transforming this approach into a data-driven endeavor. Machine learning algorithms can now process vast datasets, identifying genetic patterns and predicting how these patterns influence various traits. This computational power enables breeders to make informed decisions that steer the course of animal health over generations.

Consider the case of canine hip dysplasia, a common genetic disorder that plagues many dog breeds, causing pain and mobility issues. With the integration of AI, breeders can now identify genetic markers linked to this condition with greater accuracy. Predictive models analyze DNA sequences to assess the likelihood of offspring inheriting these markers. This level of precision allows breeders to select parent pairs that minimize the risk of dysplasia, effectively reducing its prevalence over time.

The process begins with comprehensive genomic sequencing, collecting genetic information from a variety of animals. Once the data is gathered, AI algorithms sift through it, identifying correlations and patterns that may not be discernible to the human eye. These insights are pivotal in understanding the complex relationships between different genes and their impact on health. For example, researchers may discover that a particular gene associated with coat color also plays a role in immune system function, opening avenues for breeding strategies that enhance not just aesthetic traits but also overall well-being.

AI's role in veterinary genomics is not confined to disease prevention. It also extends to enhancing desirable traits, such as improved fertility, faster growth rates, or better adaptation to environmental conditions. By understanding the genetic foundation of such traits, breeders can tailor their programs to produce animals that thrive in specific conditions, thereby fostering sustainable practices in agriculture and conservation.

Moreover, AI facilitates cross-species comparisons, allowing insights gained from one animal group to be applied to another, benefiting a wide array of species. For instance, genetic research in cattle may shed light on similar issues in other livestock, enhancing breeding strategies across the board. This cross-pollination of data and techniques stands to revolutionize how we approach animal health on a global scale.

Of course, with great power comes great responsibility. As AI continues to advance, it is crucial to balance technological capabilities with ethical considerations. Breeders and scientists must wield AI's power to promote animal welfare, ensuring that breeding practices enhance quality of life rather than prioritizing commercial or aesthetic preferences. Collaborations among geneticists, veterinarians, and AI professionals are essential to navigate these complex moral landscapes.

The dynamic nature of AI in veterinary genomics also enhances our ability to respond quickly to emerging health threats. In the past, addressing a newly identified genetic disorder might have taken decades of research and trial and error. Today, AI can accelerate this process, providing rapid assessments and potential solutions. This agility is particularly important as we face a future with shifting environmental conditions and evolving disease landscapes.

Another transformative aspect of AI in this field is its educational potential. Veterinarians and breeders can utilize AI tools to gain a deeper understanding of genetics and genomics, empowering them to apply these insights in practical settings. By demystifying the genetic underpinnings of animal health, AI fosters a culture of informed decision-making that benefits both animals and the professionals who care for them.

The integration of AI into breeding practices ultimately represents a holistic approach to animal health. It encourages a shift away from focusing solely on individual traits towards considering an animal's complete genetic profile. This broad perspective helps ensure that improvements in certain traits do not come at the expense of other important aspects of health or behavior, promoting balanced and sustainable breeding outcomes.

Looking ahead, the potential of AI in veterinary genomics appears boundless. Advances in deep learning and neural networks promise to unveil even more complex relationships within genetic data. As these technologies evolve, so too will our ability to cultivate healthier animal populations, capable of adapting to the challenges of a changing world.

In conclusion, the intersection of AI and veterinary genomics offers a powerful toolkit for improving animal health through informed breeding practices. By harnessing the computational might of AI, we gain the ability to predict, prevent, and mitigate genetic disorders while fostering desirable traits that align with both environmental demands and ethical standards. As we continue to explore this exciting frontier, collaboration remains key, ensuring that innovation in genomics serves the well-being of all creatures great and small.

Chapter 17:
AI in End-of-Life Care

In the realm of veterinary medicine, AI is carving out a compassionate path in end-of-life care, profoundly transforming the way we support animals and their owners during this sensitive time. Imagine a realm where technology doesn't replace the tender human touch but enhances it, providing insights that help veterinarians make informed, empathetic decisions. AI solutions are being developed to offer predictive analytics that forewarn caregivers about an animal's declining health, ensuring that timely and dignified care is possible. These innovations extend beyond mere data; they encompass emotional support tools for grieving pet owners, suggesting personalized coping strategies and memorial ideas. As AI continues to evolve, its role in end-of-life care promises not only to ease suffering but also to foster a shared journey of compassion and understanding between technology, veterinarians, and the families they serve.

Compassionate AI Solutions

In the realm of end-of-life care, the application of artificial intelligence is not just about employing advanced technology; it's about enriching the emotional journey for both animals and their humans. AI solutions tailored for this critical phase promise more than efficiency; they promise empathy, understanding, and grace. Indeed, integrating AI into the end-of-life process could genuinely transform an oft-difficult experience, offering solace to those managing the departure of their beloved animal companions.

One way compassionate AI solutions are shaping end-of-life care is through sophisticated predictive analytics. By analyzing health data over time, AI systems can forecast the decline of a pet's health, providing veterinarians and owners with a clearer timeline of what to expect. This predictive capability allows for better advance care planning, ensuring that appropriate measures and comforts are provided at the right time. It shifts the narrative from reactive to proactive care, granting families the chance to emotionally prepare and make the most of the remaining time.

The ability to predict and understand a pet's health trajectory opens up opportunities for personalized pain management. AI-driven applications can analyze behavioral data to assess discomfort and recommend adjustments to treatment plans. This kind of tailored approach ensures that an animal's last days are as painless and dignified as possible. By minimizing suffering, these systems embody a deep sense of compassion embedded within their algorithms, aligning technology with the humane aspects of veterinary care.

Moreover, AI applications facilitate better communication between veterinarians and pet owners, which is crucial during the sensitive phase of end-of-life care. Chatbots and AI-powered consultation platforms can address common concerns or queries outside regular office hours, offering reassurance and guidance. These tools provide a channel for immediate support, helping to ease the emotional burden on pet owners facing challenging decisions and moments.

Beyond predictive analytics and communication tools, AI-enabled devices are enhancing remote monitoring capabilities. Wearable technologies that track vital signs and movement patterns can send real-time data to veterinarians. This capability means that any significant changes in an animal's condition can be detected promptly, allowing for immediate intervention or the adjustment of care strategies. Such responsiveness not only supports the animal's well-being but also gives owners peace of mind knowing that their pet is being closely monitored, even from afar.

The emotional support provided by AI companions is another fascinating development in end-of-life care. Virtual assistants and chatbots designed with soothing human-like interactions can engage with pet owners during lonely or distressing times. These platforms can provide empathetic listening, share supportive resources, or simply remind them of the next steps in the care plan. By offering this emotional bolster, AI creates an additional layer of comfort and partnership during a profoundly personal journey.

Importantly, AI systems don't operate in isolation. They integrate seamlessly with the compassionate care regimen provided by veterinarians, aligning data-driven insights with human empathy. This synergy between technology and personal care helps to tailor the emotional and practical aspects of end-of-life management, making each case unique and personalized. Ultimately, while AI aids in making informed decisions, it is the human touch that remains pivotal in delivering the heartfelt elements of care.

AI also plays a role in honoring the life of the pet, a crucial part of the grieving process. Through technologies such as digital memory books and remembrance videos generated using AI, pet owners can cherish and revisit beautiful moments shared with their animals. These memories can then be easily personalized, offering a touching tribute to the unique bond between pet and owner. This digital commemoration can be an integral part of healing, providing a medium to celebrate life rather than just mourn its passing.

As AI continues to refine its role in veterinary medicine, incorporating artificial moral and ethical guidelines becomes necessary to ensure that compassionate care remains the priority. The goal is not just to increase efficiency but to harness technology to enhance emotional intelligence within care. AI systems need to be designed with empathy as a core feature, balancing their analytical prowess with sensitivity to human emotions and cultural contexts.

At the intersection of technology and compassion, we find transformative potential for veterinary end-of-life care. By fostering an alliance between veterinarians, tech developers, and animal owners, the field can ensure that AI solutions continue to evolve in ways that honor the life and dignity of animals. This collaborative approach will ultimately further the mission of providing gentle and respectful care when it is needed most. Through compassionate AI, the future of end-of-life care in veterinary medicine promises to be not just advanced, but truly humane.

Supporting Animals and Owners

End-of-life care for pets is an emotionally charged journey where empathy and support play crucial roles. This period, however, also poses challenges that can greatly benefit from advancements in artificial intelligence (AI). By offering solutions that blend technology with compassion, AI helps veterinarians, pet owners, and animals navigate this difficult time with empathy, precision, and sensitivity.

AI-driven systems offer tools for timely decision-making by analyzing data and predicting possible complications, which helps in designing personalized care pathways for animals approaching the end of life. These systems provide veterinarians with insights that enable them to suggest the most humane approaches tailored to each animal's unique needs and conditions. Consequently, animals can receive care that minimizes suffering and enhances their quality of life in their final days.

For pet owners, AI can serve as a valuable ally in making informed decisions. It's not just about clinical recommendations but providing a comprehensive understanding of the pet's condition through accessible platforms that illustrate scenarios and potential outcomes. AI's predictive capabilities offer owners a glimpse into future possibilities, helping in preparing emotionally and practically for the steps ahead.

Advanced AI systems drive innovations in communication between veterinary teams and the pet owners they serve, allowing for more nuanced discussions at a time of often heightened emotion and stress. Integrating AI into management systems enables the tracking of an animal's health metrics in real time, thus fostering open and continuous dialogue between owners and care providers.

Emotional support is another area where AI shows promising potential. While the touching presence of a pet can't be replaced, AI technologies are developing capabilities to recognize and respond to the emotional states of owners. Compassionate virtual assistants, armed with patterns from years of data analyzing human and animal interaction, might offer supportive suggestions or gently remind caregivers of routines that can bring comfort and familiarity to pets.

Significantly, AI also aids in understanding the grieving process that owners face. Algorithms designed to monitor social and digital interactions can gently evaluate the owner's emotional well-being and can direct them to resources or social support networks if needed. Offering such mental health support ensures that the entire family unit—human and animal alike—is supported through these challenging end-of-life matters.

AI-enriched memory preservation services provide opportunities for extending the legacy of the departed pet. They enable owners to create digital memorials that not only celebrate memories through photos, videos, and stories but also offer a platform for shared grief. By assisting in these imperceptibly small yet profound ways, AI can honor the intangible bond shared between owners and their beloved pets.

End-of-life decisions are among the toughest that pet owners face. AI helps facilitate those decisions by offering evidence-based recommendations while honoring the emotional nuances involved. Mechanical or distant these machines are not, yet they bridge the knowledge gap that often leaves many owners feeling unprepared to make these decisions amid sorrow.

Further integration of AI into support systems promises to humanize and elevate the care animals receive during their final journey. As AI continues to evolve, its ability to deepen the bonds between pets and their owners, even at the end of life, is becoming increasingly clear. What's unmistakable is the transformative potential AI holds in ensuring that as we bid farewell to our pets, we do so with grace, empathy, and honor.

By demystifying complex medical information and providing a channel for emotional support, AI arms veterinarians and pet owners with the tools necessary to approach end-of-life care with confidence and care. Supporting animals and their owners means acknowledging the profound connection they share and aspiring to maintain that bond with dignity until the very end.

Chapter 18:
Legal and Regulatory Aspects of AI

The rapidly advancing integration of artificial intelligence in veterinary medicine offers tremendous potential, but it also comes with a complex web of legal and regulatory challenges that animal healthcare providers must navigate. As veterinarians increasingly rely on AI technologies to diagnose, treat, and monitor animal health, ensuring compliance with existing regulations and understanding emerging legal frameworks becomes crucial. These regulations are designed not just to protect animal welfare and privacy, but to ensure that AI applications in veterinary settings maintain ethical standards and transparency. Balancing innovation with compliance involves understanding both national and international standards, which can differ significantly in scope and detail. As AI technology evolves, so too do the regulatory landscapes, prompting ongoing dialogue between tech developers, veterinarians, regulatory bodies, and policymakers. Compliance ensures not only legality but also builds trust with pet owners and the public, underscoring a commitment to responsible, accountable use of these transformative tools in enhancing animal care.

Navigating AI Regulations

The rapid evolution of artificial intelligence (AI) in veterinary medicine presents exciting opportunities alongside significant regulatory challenges. Navigating AI regulations is pivotal for ensuring that innovations not only enhance animal healthcare but also comply with legal standards. In a field as dynamic as veterinary medicine, where technology intersects with ethics and patient care, understanding and adapting to these regulations is crucial.

AI regulations on a global scale vary widely, influenced by differing legal frameworks and cultural attitudes towards technology. In the United States, for instance, veterinary applications of AI fall under the purview of the Food and Drug Administration (FDA), particularly when AI technologies are integrated into medical devices used for diagnosing or treating animals. The FDA's guidelines emphasize ensuring the safety, effectiveness, and quality of AI tools, which requires rigorous testing and validation before they can be deployed in clinical settings.

Understanding these regulations involves grasping a variety of concepts, from the classification of AI technologies to compliance with data protection laws like the General Data Protection Regulation (GDPR) in Europe. The GDPR emphasizes the need for transparency and accountability in handling personal data, which includes animal data collected through AI devices. This regulation poses unique challenges for AI-driven veterinary practices, especially given the global nature of animal healthcare services and cross-border research collaborations.

Veterinarians and AI developers often face a labyrinth of legal and regulatory issues. The classification of AI systems is a starting point: are they considered medical devices or tools intended for research? This distinction influences the regulatory pathway and the extent of oversight required. For example, AI algorithms used to interpret radiographic images may be classified as medical devices, necessitating rigorous validation processes similar to those applied to traditional diagnostic equipment.

Additionally, intellectual property rights and liability questions further complicate the regulatory landscape. As AI systems increasingly make independent decisions, determining who holds responsibility and liability becomes complex. Is it the developer who designed the algorithm, the veterinarian interpreting the results, or the clinic's management? These questions underscore the need for clear legal frameworks that account for the multifaceted nature of AI technologies.

The veterinary community must also consider how regulations might evolve as AI technologies advance. Adaptive regulatory frameworks that keep pace with technological innovation are essential. For instance, the integration of machine learning into regulatory protocols offers the potential for more dynamic oversight, allowing regulations to adjust as AI systems learn and improve over time. However, such adaptability requires a deep-rooted collaboration between tech developers, veterinarians, and regulators.

Regulatory compliance isn't merely about meeting current standards; it involves anticipating and shaping future policies. Proactive engagement with regulatory bodies can facilitate the development of guidelines that are both robust and flexible. Veterinary professionals can play a pivotal role, offering insights into practical challenges and ethical considerations that tech developers and legislators might overlook. This collaborative effort ensures that the regulations imposed are grounded in the realities of veterinary practice and animal welfare.

Moreover, international cooperation in setting AI standards for veterinary medicine can drive harmonization of regulations. This harmonization is crucial in an interconnected world where knowledge sharing and medical interventions often cross borders. Global coalitions such as the International Coalition for Animal Immunosuppressive Drug Approval (ICADA) advocate for consistent regulatory standards and help streamline the process for innovative treatments, including those that leverage AI.

Ethical considerations are intertwined with regulatory aspects. As AI systems become more autonomous, the potential for ethical dilemmas increases. Developers and practitioners must ensure that AI-driven techniques respect the intrinsic value of animal life, adhere to the principles of animal welfare, and maintain trust with pet owners. Ethical guidelines complement legal regulations, offering a framework for dealing with potential issues of consent, particularly when owners rely on AI tools to make critical decisions about their pet's health care.

Training and education play a critical role in enabling veterinarians and their teams to navigate AI regulations effectively. Understanding regulatory requirements and keeping abreast of changes can be as crucial as mastering the technical aspects of AI technologies themselves. Continuing education courses, workshops, and certification programs focused on the legal and regulatory aspects of AI are vital resources for fostering expertise and compliance within the veterinary community.

The financial implications of regulatory compliance cannot be overlooked. Developing AI tools that meet stringent regulatory standards often requires significant investment in testing, validation, and documentation. These costs can be a barrier to innovation, especially for smaller veterinary practices or startups entering the AI field. However, investing in compliance can ultimately protect these entities from legal repercussions and build credibility with clients, regulators, and the broader public.

In conclusion, navigating AI regulations in veterinary medicine is an intricate process that demands careful consideration of legal, ethical, and practical elements. While the challenges are substantial, they are surmountable through collaboration, education, and proactive engagement with regulatory agencies. As AI continues to transform animal healthcare, aligning innovation with compliance will ensure that technological advancements translate into tangible benefits for pets, livestock, and wildlife, fostering a future where AI and veterinary medicine work in concert to elevate animal health and welfare.

Ensuring Compliance in Veterinary Care

In the rapidly evolving world of artificial intelligence, veterinary care must navigate a complex web of legal and regulatory frameworks. These frameworks ensure that while benefiting from cutting-edge AI technologies, high ethical standards and legal compliance are maintained. The journey begins with understanding the legal landscape governing AI use in animal healthcare, which balances innovation with the need for responsibility and safety.

One of the primary goals for veterinarians using AI is to stay within legal boundaries. Unlike other fields, veterinary medicine involves diverse species, each with unique considerations and needs. Thus, laws and regulations must be adaptable. Veterinarians must continuously update their knowledge about these regulations so they can effectively integrate AI technologies into their practices without running afoul of legal entities. This educational endeavor requires commitment, not just from veterinarians but also from associations that govern veterinary medicine worldwide.

At the heart of ensuring compliance is the concept of informed consent. With AI systems assisting in diagnostics or treatment, veterinarians must clearly communicate the role and limitations of AI tools to pet owners. This transparency fosters trust, allowing owners to make informed decisions about their pets' healthcare. It also serves as a legal safeguard, ensuring that all parties comprehend the extent and limitations of AI involvement in veterinary care.

Moreover, data protection and privacy laws form a crucial component of AI compliance in veterinary settings. AI systems rely heavily on data, including sensitive health information. Veterinarians need to navigate these regulations carefully, ensuring that data is collected, stored, and utilized following applicable privacy laws. Adopting robust data protection protocols not only protects the business legally but also reassures clients that their pets' information is securely handled.

To facilitate compliance, various governing bodies have been working to develop guidelines and standards for AI use. These standards aim to harmonize the application of AI across veterinary practices, ensuring that all practitioners adhere to a consistent framework of ethical and legal principles. Such efforts contribute to a unified approach, helping veterinarians around the world leverage AI technology effectively and responsibly.

One of the significant challenges in this domain is keeping pace with the rapid advancement of AI technologies. As AI continues to develop, so must the legal frameworks that regulate its use. This is not a simple task, as legislation typically lags behind technology. Nevertheless, proactive engagement from the veterinary community with regulators can help bridge this gap, ensuring that the laws that do exist reflect the realities of modern practice and technology.

International collaboration is another vital element in harmonizing regulations. Veterinary care is a global field, with practitioners often relying on technologies developed in other countries. Aligning international standards helps ensure consistency across borders, reducing the potential for confusion or exploitation of regulatory loopholes. Such agreements foster an environment where AI can thrive while still protecting animal welfare and maintaining ethical boundaries.

Professional development also plays a crucial role in maintaining compliance. As AI becomes more integral to veterinary practice, ongoing training and education become indispensable. Continued education programs focused on emerging legal issues, ethical considerations, and technological advancements ensure that veterinarians remain knowledgeable. They can then adapt to evolving legal landscapes, safeguarding their practices and their patients.

Insurance companies are showing growing interest in AI compliance as well. As AI plays a larger role in veterinary decision-making processes, insurance companies need to assess the implications for risk and coverage. This may require new insurance policies or the adaptation of existing ones to better address the nuances related to AI-driven treatments and diagnostics.

Furthermore, ethical considerations cannot be ignored when discussing legal compliance in AI-enhanced veterinary care. Ethical AI use involves ensuring that AI tools are utilized to enhance, not replace, the judgment and empathy inherent in veterinary care. Compliance in this context means adhering not just to the letter of the law but also to the spirit, ensuring AI serves as a tool for better care rather than a threat to the human-animal bond.

Lastly, veterinary practices must develop internal compliance strategies tailored to their specific needs. Establishing defined protocols for integrating AI tools, monitoring their performance, and regularly reviewing their legal obligations ensures ongoing compliance. Regular audits can also help practices identify potential areas of non-compliance, allowing them to address these proactively and mitigate risks.

Overall, ensuring compliance in veterinary care is not a static goal but an ongoing process. It requires a comprehensive approach involving education, the development of internal policies, international collaboration, and a proactive relationship with regulatory bodies. By embracing these, the veterinary community can continue to benefit from AI's myriad advantages while maintaining the highest standards of legal and ethical practice.

Chapter 19:
Financial Impact of AI on Veterinary Practices

The financial landscape of veterinary practices is being reshaped by artificial intelligence, infusing remarkable efficiency and potential profit enhancements. In today's rapidly evolving market, AI has become an integral player, optimizing operations from scheduling and resource allocation to precise diagnostics and personalized treatment plans. This technological infusion often translates into cost savings, as streamlined processes reduce time and resource consumption, allowing veterinary practitioners to maximize patient care and revenue streams. However, the financial benefits of AI extend beyond mere operational efficiency. As AI-driven solutions foster accurate diagnoses and treatments, they enhance service quality, building client trust and potentially expanding client bases. While the initial investment in AI tools demands thoughtful financial planning, the prospect of increased profitability presents compelling opportunities for clinics ready to embrace this transformation. Moreover, partnerships and funding initiatives are increasingly available, offering veterinarians the financial leverage they need to implement these advanced technologies. Thus, AI not only promises a healthier future for animals but also positions veterinary practices on a trajectory toward enhanced economic sustainability.

Cost-Benefit Analysis

The integration of artificial intelligence into veterinary practices presents a multifaceted opportunity that demands a thorough cost-benefit analysis. For veterinarians, it's not just a question of financial investment but a puzzle that requires balancing new technologies with traditional veterinary methods. The promise AI offers is significant, but so are the challenges and potential risks involved. This section will delve into both sides, offering insights for practitioners considering the incorporation of AI into their clinics.

On the cost side, the initial investment is a predominant concern. AI systems, particularly those involving machine learning algorithms and complex data management tools, often require substantial upfront funds. Veterinarians may need to invest in new hardware, software, and staff training to leverage these technologies effectively. Additionally, the ongoing costs related to software updates, system maintenance, and potential data storage solutions must be factored into budget considerations.

Beyond direct financial investments, there are indirect costs such as the time needed for implementation and the risk of potential disruption to existing workflows. Transitioning to AI-enhanced systems isn't without its learning curve. Veterinary staff must be adept with new interfaces, necessitating training periods that could initially slow down operations. These hidden costs can be significant and must be carefully evaluated.

Despite these costs, the benefits AI can bring to veterinary practices are compelling. For instance, AI-driven diagnostics have been shown to improve accuracy and speed in identifying diseases, ultimately leading to more effective treatments. This capability not only enhances patient outcomes but also increases client satisfaction. Happy clients are likely to return and recommend the practice, potentially driving up revenue in the long run.

The automation of repetitive tasks is another benefit AI can provide, allowing vet technicians and doctors to focus on more complex and engaging aspects of care. By reducing the burden of routine tasks, practices can optimize their labor resources, potentially lowering operational costs over time. Furthermore, AI systems can operate round-the-clock, providing data insights and alerts on patient health without the need for human oversight.

AI's predictive capabilities can also be advantageous. For example, predictive analytics can assist in inventory management, helping practices maintain optimal stock levels of medications and supplies while reducing waste and storage costs. This, in turn, leads to smarter business operations and improved financial efficiency.

Long-term, adopting AI could position veterinary practices ahead of industry trends. As more clinics embrace these technologies, those who don't risk falling behind both functionally and competitively. Early adopters might find themselves at the forefront of innovation, becoming leaders in a tech-driven market. Keeping up-to-date with the latest AI advancements could provide a competitive edge that attracts tech-savvy clients interested in cutting-edge veterinary care for their pets.

However, the financial implications go beyond direct services and operations. AI can open new revenue streams through data-driven services, such as customized nutrition plans or advanced health monitoring subscriptions for pet owners. These additional services could become significant income sources, augmenting traditional offerings and expanding the practice's market reach.

It's also worth noting the potential for AI to aid in compliance with veterinary regulations. Automated reporting and monitoring can ensure that practices meet industry standards with greater ease, potentially reducing the risk of costly penalties associated with compliance issues. By ensuring practices run smoothly and according to regulations, AI can mitigate the financial risks associated with legal liabilities.

The decision to integrate AI into a veterinary practice ultimately hinges on whether the expected benefits outweigh the costs. Every practice has its unique set of circumstances, so a one-size-fits-all approach doesn't work here. Some clinics may find immediate advantages, particularly those with a strong tech orientation or a client base that values innovation. Others might need to proceed with caution, evaluating incremental solutions rather than a full-scale transformation.

As the field continues to evolve, veterinary professionals must engage in ongoing learning and adaptability. Staying informed about AI trends, advancements, and best practices becomes crucial. Through professional networks, seminars, and workshops, vets can stay at the forefront of AI utilizations in their field, ensuring they reap the benefits while managing the costs effectively.

While significant investments in AI are daunting, it bears noting that technology often decreases in cost as it matures and becomes more widely adopted. With strategic planning, careful evaluation, and measured implementation, the integration of AI doesn't have to be financially prohibitive. Strategic investments today can lead to substantial long-term gains, making AI an invaluable tool for the modern veterinarian, tech enthusiast, or animal advocate.

Funding and Investment Opportunities

For veterinarians eyeing the horizons shaped by artificial intelligence, the financial landscape isn't just about managing costs—it's about unlocking new avenues of growth and innovation. The wave of AI isn't merely a trend; it's a transformative force demanding strategic investment. But where do these opportunities lie, and how can veterinary practices capitalize on them?

Firstly, understanding the ecosystem of funding opportunities for AI-driven interventions is pivotal. The intersection of AI and veterinary medicine has caught the attention of government bodies, private investors, and tech companies. Such stakeholders recognize the potential of AI to address some of the pressing challenges in animal health care, prompting them to open their coffers. Government grants specifically aimed at integrating technology into veterinary practices can provide the requisite boost to initiate AI projects. Moreover, tech companies often offer partnership opportunities or seed funding to develop AI applications that enhance their suite of solutions. Thus, staying informed about these sources of funding is crucial for practices aiming to integrate AI.

Private equity firms and venture capitalists are also showing increasing interest in the veterinary sector, drawn by the notion of unlocking unprecedented efficiencies through AI. These investors are keen to support practices that are willing to explore AI interventions, from diagnostic tools to predictive analytics. By presenting a solid business plan that delineates the potential return on investment, veterinary practices can attract funds that help them leapfrog traditional methods. The key here is to demonstrate how AI can lead to cost savings, improved customer service, or novel revenue streams, ensuring that investors are seeing a tangible value proposition.

Beyond seeking external funding, investing internally in AI adoption can lead to financial benefits that far outstrip initial costs. Practices that allocate resources to train their team and overhaul their infrastructure to accommodate AI solutions often see a significant reduction in operational inefficiencies. Such investments can manifest in faster processing of diagnostic results or more precise prescription and treatment plans, ultimately enhancing the revenue cycle by offering better customer satisfaction and loyalty.

Additionally, as AI solutions become more refined, the potential for reducing veterinary practice overheads becomes more pronounced. AI tools can automate administrative tasks, reduce staff workloads, and minimize errors associated with human data entry. These efficiencies not only save costs on staffing but also open the doors to expanding the services without proportional increases in overheads. This creates a solid argument for internal reinvestment in AI tools and showcases a pathway that veterinary practices can follow to expand their service offerings without incurring prohibitive costs.

It's also worth considering the insurance industry's response to AI in veterinary practices. Companies are beginning to offer discounts to practices that implement reliable AI systems, particularly those that contribute to risk management or enhance care quality. Insurance incentives can thus play a critical role in offsetting the financial burden of AI adoption, serving as yet another funding stream that practices can leverage while transitioning to more technologically advanced operations.

Practices should not overlook the potential for community and client engagement to translate into investment opportunities. By involving clients in the journey towards AI adoption, especially through educational workshops or demonstration events, practices can inspire contributions from patrons who are willing to sponsor advancements in technology that promise enhanced care for their pets. This sense of community investment not only fosters a deeper bond with clients but also helps spread the financial burden of technology adoption over a larger base.

The strategic investment in AI isn't just about finances; it's also about future-proofing veterinary practices. As AI becomes more entrenched in everyday operations, early adopters are likely to have a significant competitive advantage. By seizing funding and investment opportunities now, practices can position themselves as leaders in a rapidly evolving field, ready to meet the demands of an increasingly tech-savvy clientele. In doing so, they're not only hedging against obsolescence but also aligning with a future where AI aids in providing top-tier animal care.

Finally, capturing these opportunities requires a shift in mindset—from seeing AI as an overhead to viewing it as an investment. It's about making informed choices that blend technological potential with financial foresight. As AI continues to revolutionize the veterinary industry, practices that harness funding and investment opportunities intelligently will not only enhance their bottom line but also redefine the standards of care they deliver. In this thrilling convergence of technology and animal health, the possibilities are as boundless as the imagination of those willing to invest in the future.

Chapter 20:
Case Studies in AI-Enhanced Veterinary Care

In recent years, the world of veterinary medicine has witnessed remarkable strides thanks to AI's transformative power, illustrated vividly through diverse case studies. Across varied settings, from bustling urban clinics to remote wildlife reserves, AI's integration into routine practice is reshaping healthcare delivery for animals. Consider a scenario where AI algorithms, working seamlessly with imaging technologies, significantly reduced the diagnosis time for a rare condition in a golden retriever. This isn't an isolated success. In another example, algorithms tailored diet plans for zoo elephants, improving their health and behavioral patterns. These stories showcase not only technological prowess but the profound impacts on animal well-being. Through these real-world applications, veterinarians embrace AI as a catalyst for positive change, enhancing their ability to provide precise, compassionate care. The lessons learned highlight AI's potential to bridge gaps in veterinary expertise, offering insights into where it's most effective and flagging areas needing caution and further development.

Success Stories from the Field

The transformative power of artificial intelligence (AI) in veterinary medicine is best illustrated through real-world success stories. These stories not only exemplify the groundbreaking achievements of AI-enhanced veterinary care but also offer a glimpse into the future of animal healthcare. From bustling urban clinics to the open plains of wildlife reserves, AI has emerged as a guiding force for veterinarians worldwide.

In a thriving metropolitan animal hospital in New York, Dr. Sophia Alvarez and her team have witnessed a revolution in diagnostic accuracy thanks to AI. A busy practice, they see countless pets with varying ailments each day. One case stands out—a chocolate Labrador named Max, who was suffering from unexplained weight loss and lethargy. Traditional lab tests offered no clear answers. However, incorporating AI tools for image analysis uncovered a rare parasite infection within hours, a diagnosis that would have taken weeks through conventional methods. Max's swift recovery was a testament to the power of AI in providing rapid and precise diagnostics.

Across the globe in rural Kenya, AI systems are making a significant impact on wildlife conservation efforts. At the renowned Amboseli Elephant Research Project, researchers paired AI with drone technology to monitor elephant populations more effectively. This innovative approach has improved tracking, leading to better protection strategies against poaching. Data from AI-driven analysis has helped identify migratory patterns and herd behavior, offering insights that are crucial for conservationists. As a result, elephant populations in the region have shown promising signs of recovery.

Meanwhile, in Florida, an AI-driven telemedicine platform is bridging the gap between busy pet owners and veterinary professionals. A high-volume clinic managed by Dr. Jeff Thompson has successfully integrated teleconsultations with AI assistance, significantly reducing wait times for pet care. For pet owners like Sarah, whose cat Whiskers was showing signs of respiratory distress, it provided peace of mind and immediate action. The AI-assisted consultations enabled precise assessments and timely interventions, enhancing client satisfaction and improving animal outcomes.

AI has also proven invaluable in revolutionizing preventive health strategies. At a cutting-edge veterinary practice in California, Dr. Emily Chen employs predictive analytics powered by AI to foresee potential health issues in her clients' pets. For instance, analyzing diet, exercise habits, and genetic predispositions has allowed the practice to identify early signs of diabetes in cats. Tailored intervention plans have resulted in healthier, happier pets and significantly decreased complications, proving that prevention is indeed better than cure.

The veterinary world is also seeing AI-driven success stories in animal behavior analysis. In the bustling city of Tokyo, a pioneering project by behavioral experts has employed AI to interpret dog behaviors and optimize training methods. Using a combination of video analysis and machine learning, they've trained service dogs more effectively, benefiting communities with special needs. Dogs trained with this AI assistance have exhibited enhanced skills, leading to life-changing support for their handlers and families.

In farms sprawling across the Midwest, AI technologies in precision agriculture are helping veterinarians and farmers manage livestock health better. Farm operations utilizing AI for predictive health management have seen remarkable improvements in livestock well-being and productivity. By detecting subtle changes in behavior and physical activity, AI systems alert caretakers to potential issues long before they become severe. This has resulted in fewer illnesses and improved overall animal welfare, showcasing the economic and ethical benefits of AI integration.

In another case, a specialty referral center in Sydney adopted AI-enhanced surgical techniques to perform intricate procedures with remarkable precision. Here, the AI-assisted robotic system worked alongside veterinary surgeons to execute complex hip surgeries on dogs with a history of trauma. The outcomes were astounding, with reduced recovery times and exceptional post-operative results. The integration of robotics not only improved surgical outcomes but also enhanced surgeon confidence and efficiency.

The scope of AI in veterinary medicine extends beyond individual cases, reaching into collaborative research projects as well. At a reputable veterinary school in London, AI has facilitated breakthroughs in genomic research, fast-tracking studies that could have taken years. This has led to new insights into animal diseases and improved breeding programs, offering long-term health benefits for diverse species.

These success stories demonstrate a paradigm shift, as AI continues to redefine the landscape of veterinary care. However, the potential of AI in animal healthcare is far from fully realized. As technologies evolve, the promise of more success stories is inevitable, painting a brighter future for veterinarians, pet owners, and animals alike.

The journey of AI in veterinary care, much like the stories aforementioned, is filled with challenges and triumphs. With each success story, whether in urban clinics or wild savannas, AI not only enhances veterinary expertise but also fosters a new bond between humans and animals. As we look ahead, these tales of success fuel our passion for innovation and commitment to advancing animal health in every corner of the globe.

Lessons Learned from Implementation

The integration of artificial intelligence into veterinary care has been a transformative journey, marked with significant achievements and valuable insights. As veterinary practices embraced AI technologies, initial expectations were high, driven by the potential to revolutionize diagnostics, treatment personalization, and overall animal care.

However, the path wasn't straightforward, and each step revealed critical lessons, shaping the future trajectory of AI in the field.

One of the primary lessons learned was the importance of adaptability. Veterinary practitioners discovered that AI systems, despite their potential, require continuous refinement and adaptation to meet the unique needs of different animal species. Unlike human medicine, where AI applications might find a common ground, veterinary care must account for the diversity of species, each with its distinct physiological and behavioral characteristics. Veterinarians realized the necessity of collaborating closely with AI developers to tailor technologies that accommodate this diversity.

Furthermore, the implementation of AI underscored the significance of data quality. AI's effectiveness heavily relies on robust, accurate data to train algorithms, yet many veterinary practices struggled with fragmented or incomplete datasets. This realization emphasized the need for better data management practices and collaboration across institutions to develop comprehensive datasets that ensure AI models are both reliable and generalizable. It became clear that investing in data infrastructure and standardization practices was essential for harnessing AI's full capability.

Another critical insight gained from implementing AI in veterinary care was the necessity for ongoing education and training. Many practitioners initially faced a steep learning curve, as AI technologies introduced new concepts and platforms that were unfamiliar. Veterinary professionals recognized the importance of continuous education and professional development to stay abreast of AI advancements. Establishing regular training sessions and workshops became a priority, ensuring that the workforce could effectively utilize AI tools and processes, thereby enhancing their confidence and proficiency in AI applications.

Communication emerged as a crucial component in the successful deployment of AI systems. Bridging the gap between AI developers and veterinarians required fostering effective channels of communication. Misalignment in understanding each other's needs and capabilities often led to misunderstandings or under-utilization of AI technology. Transparent and open dialogues between the two domains became imperative, not just in the initial stages of development but throughout the implementation phase, facilitating an environment where innovations could thrive and evolve.

In addition to technical and operational adjustments, ethical considerations became a focal point. Veterinarians grappled with questions about data privacy, informed consent, and the responsible use of AI-driven insights in diagnosis and treatment. Lessons learned from ethical dilemmas emphasized the need for establishing clear guidelines and frameworks addressing these concerns. By proactively engaging with ethical principles, veterinarians can ensure that the integration of AI aligns with professional values and public trust, maintaining the welfare of animals and the confidence of their owners.

Economic realities also shaped the understanding of AI applications in veterinary settings. While AI can offer cost-effective solutions over time, the initial investment in technology, training, and infrastructure posed economic challenges for some practices. Learning how to strategically allocate resources, assess financial benefits, and explore funding opportunities proved vital for sustainable AI adoption. Practices were encouraged to conduct thorough cost-benefit analyses before implementation, evaluating the long-term financial impacts alongside potential improvements to care quality.

Beyond the walls of veterinary clinics, the implementation highlighted the impact of AI on the broader ecosystem of animal care. The technologies facilitated enhanced collaborations with research institutions, zoos, and conservation organizations, leading to interdisciplinary partnerships. This broader network fostered sharing of knowledge and innovations, propelling the veterinary field into a collaborative future where AI applications extend beyond individual practices to global animal health and conservation efforts.

Importantly, AI's presence in veterinary care taught professionals about the evolving dynamics of human-animal interaction facilitated by technology. Practitioners found that AI-enabled tools could enhance their understanding of patient behavior and health trends, providing deeper insights that enriched the veterinarian-animal bond. This new dimension of care emphasized the power of empathy and human expertise in tandem with AI capabilities, reinforcing the notion that technology serves as a complement, not a replacement, to the compassionate care that defines veterinary medicine.

As AI systems matured within veterinary practices, unexpected results and creative problem-solving emerged, revealing the flexibility and innovative potential inherent in AI technology. Veterinarians witnessed AI's ability to adapt and provide novel solutions to complex challenges, inspiring a shift in mindset from traditional practices to a more experimental, iterative approach to animal healthcare. Embracing this mindset encouraged not only technological innovation but also cultural shifts towards resilience and openness to change within veterinary teams.

Finally, the implementation phase brought to light the role of community engagement and public perception in successful AI integration. Veterinarians understood the need for transparent communication with clients, educating them about AI's role and benefits in treatment plans. Building trust and addressing any misconceptions became integral to fostering a supportive community that views AI advancements as allies in the pursuit of optimal animal health.

In conclusion, the lessons learned from implementing AI in veterinary care serve as a compass for navigating future endeavors in this dynamic field. Adaptability, communication, ethical vigilance, continuous education, and a collaborative spirit stand as pillars supporting the ongoing journey of AI-enhanced animal care. These insights pave the way for future innovations, ensuring that AI-driven solutions not only transform practices but profoundly enrich the lives of animals and their caregivers across the globe.

Chapter 21:
Future Trends in AI for Animal Health

The future of AI in animal health is poised to revolutionize the field with emerging technologies that promise unprecedented advancements. We're at the cusp of integrating AI with genomics and data analytics to anticipate health trends and personalize treatments like never before. Imagine AI algorithms that can predict disease outbreaks in livestock or diagnose rare conditions in exotic species with precision and speed. There's also growing potential in enhancing remote monitoring and telehealth services, making veterinary care more accessible to underserved areas. Over the next decade, the emphasis will likely shift towards sustainable practices, with AI driving green technologies in veterinary care and promoting eco-friendly solutions. As AI continues to evolve, the collaboration between veterinarians and AI specialists will be crucial to harness these innovations effectively, ensuring that technological advancements align with ethical considerations and the welfare of the animals we cherish. This burgeoning field offers a glimpse into a future where AI not only transforms animal healthcare but also fosters a healthier, more harmonious coexistence between humans and animals.

Emerging Technologies

The landscape of animal healthcare is being transformed by the advent of emerging technologies powered by artificial intelligence. These innovations are set to redefine how veterinarians diagnose, treat, and manage animal health. As we delve into the future trends in AI, it becomes evident that the integration of cutting-edge technologies presents both opportunities and challenges in veterinary care.

One of the most promising emerging technologies is the use of AI in imaging and diagnostics. Advanced imaging techniques, such as 3D imaging and machine learning algorithms, are enabling veterinarians to detect anomalies with unparalleled accuracy. These technologies don't just improve diagnostic capabilities; they also enhance the precision and speed of identifying health issues. By leveraging images collected from a variety of modalities, AI systems can assist in creating comprehensive health profiles for animals, leading to more accurate and timely interventions.

AI-driven biosensors are another burgeoning area with substantial implications for animal health. These tiny, intelligent sensors are capable of monitoring a range of physiological parameters in real-time, from heart rates to stress levels, which are transmitted to cloud-based AI systems for analysis. These systems can then alert veterinarians or pet owners to potential health issues before they become critical, ensuring proactive care and potentially saving lives. This technology not only benefits domestic pets but also finds significant application in monitoring wildlife and livestock health on a large scale.

The field of genomics is also witnessing a transformation through AI. By analyzing large datasets of genetic information, AI technologies are facilitating breakthroughs in understanding genetic predispositions to diseases and ideal breeding practices. Gene editing technologies, supported by AI, offer the potential to eradicate or mitigate genetic disorders in both domesticated animals and wildlife populations. This power to address health from a genetic level is setting the stage for revolutionary improvements in both treatment and preventive care.

Robotic automation in veterinary surgeries is yet another frontier where AI is making its mark. These robotic systems, equipped with precision instruments and guided by AI algorithms, offer enhanced dexterity and precision that can surpass the limitations of the human hand. The integration of these technologies reduces the likelihood of human error and improves recovery times for surgical patients.

In a similar vein, AI-powered telemedicine platforms are becoming increasingly sophisticated. These platforms allow for remote consultations and diagnostics, bridging the gap between pet owners and veterinary professionals. By extending access to high-quality veterinary care to remote areas, these platforms are democratizing animal healthcare like never before. They provide a wealth of insights into health trends across different regions, feeding back into AI systems to refine diagnostic and treatment approaches continually.

AI's role in developing smart wearable devices for animals is another exciting development. These devices track vital statistics and behavioral patterns, offering a continuous stream of data that AI can analyze to detect potential health issues. The ability to monitor animals 24/7 facilitates a deeper understanding of their health, enabling quick interventions when necessary and lending insights into preventative care strategies.

Moreover, the fusion of AI with augmented and virtual reality technologies holds great promise for veterinary education and training. These immersive experiences enable students and practitioners to gain deeper insights into complex procedures and rare conditions without the risk associated with live practice. As a result, we are seeing a new generation of veterinarians who are more prepared than ever to tackle the complexities of modern veterinary medicine.

Despite these advances, the integration of emerging technologies in animal healthcare is not without challenges. Concerns around data privacy, ethical implications of genetic modifications, and the need for regulatory frameworks to manage AI adoption are at the forefront. The veterinary profession must engage in ongoing conversations to navigate these challenges while embracing the potential that AI holds for revolutionizing animal care.

As these emerging technologies continue to evolve, their successful integration into veterinary practice hinges on collaboration. Veterinarians, AI experts, and technology developers must engage in collaborative efforts to bridge knowledge gaps and ensure the practical application of these innovations. By working together, these stakeholders can effectively navigate the complex landscape of AI in animal healthcare, ensuring that these technologies serve the best interests of both animals and their caregivers.

Looking ahead, the role of emerging technologies in veterinary medicine will only grow. As AI systems become increasingly sophisticated, their ability to transform animal healthcare becomes apparent, promising unprecedented improvements in diagnostics, treatment, and animal welfare. Embracing these changes requires a forward-thinking approach that blends technological innovation with compassionate care, setting the stage for a future where animal health continues to flourish under the guidance of intelligent machines.

Predictions for the Next Decade

The future of artificial intelligence in veterinary medicine is set to transform the landscape of animal healthcare profoundly. Looking ahead to the next decade, we can anticipate several dynamic shifts driven by technological advancements and increasing integration of AI into everyday veterinary practice. The convergence of AI with veterinary care promises to streamline operations, enhance precision in diagnostics and treatments, and ultimately, improve outcomes for animals across the globe.

One of the most compelling predictions for the future involves the increasing sophistication of AI-driven diagnostic tools. As machine learning algorithms become more refined, they're likely to surpass the limitations of current tools. Imagine a world where AI provides instant, accurate diagnoses for a wider breadth of conditions in animals, helping veterinarians not only detect existing health issues but also foresee potential ones before they manifest. This could drastically change the approach to animal health, shifting from reactive to proactive management, sparking a revolution in preventative care.

Personalized medicine, a cornerstone of human healthcare advancements, is likely to become a reality in animal health as AI tools evolve. In the coming decade, AI's ability to analyze vast amounts of genetic data rapidly will enable veterinarians to design highly customized treatment plans tailored to the unique genetic make-up and lifestyle of each animal. This precision in personalization could extend the lifespan and quality of life for pets, livestock, and wildlife.

AI's capacity to analyze and interpret complex datasets will transform the way veterinarians understand animal behavior. By utilizing behavioral data collected through AI-enabled devices, veterinary professionals will gain deeper insights than ever before. This will enhance our understanding of conditions such as anxiety or aggression in domestic pets and help manage them with greater efficacy. Imagine companions with fewer behavioral issues, thanks to the interventions developed through these insights.

Telemedicine is another field ripe for expansion over the next decade, as AI continues to break down barriers and bring veterinary care to remote regions. The ability of AI to facilitate real-time consultations and diagnoses, irrespective of geographical constraints, will likely lead to a more democratized access to veterinary care. This could be especially beneficial for rural areas and developing nations, where access is currently limited.

In terms of research and development, the next ten years could witness AI playing a pivotal role in drug discovery and veterinary medicinal advancements. By accelerating the drug development cycle,

AI might reduce costs and the time necessary to bring new treatments to market. The knock-on effect of this could be the faster availability of innovative therapeutics to treat and manage a wide variety of animal health issues.

AI technology will likely expand its influence not only in clinical settings but also on the farm. Livestock farming, pivotal to global food security, stands to gain immeasurably from AI applications. Farmers could employ AI to monitor the health and productivity of herds, optimize feed efficiency, and even predict birthing events to provide timely care reducing mortality rates. This innovation hints at a future where livestock farming is more sustainable, efficient, and ethical.

With advances in AI, a major focus will be on conservation efforts. AI's role in monitoring wildlife populations and biodiversity will become even more integral. We can expect innovations that improve the tracking of endangered species, helping conservationists assess threats more accurately and devise effective strategies. In essence, AI will serve as a crucial ally in preserving the planet's delicate ecological balance.

As these technological advancements unfold, ethical considerations surrounding the use of AI in veterinary medicine will gain prominence. The debate around data privacy, bias in AI algorithms, and the responsible use of technology in decision-making for animal health will intensify. Consequently, the next decade is likely to see a robust framework of ethical guidelines and regulations formulated to ensure AI applications in animal healthcare are equitable and responsible.

The integration of AI in veterinary medicine will also reshape the educational landscape over the coming years. By equipping future veterinarians with AI-enhanced learning tools, educational institutions will prepare them to leverage technology as an integral part of animal care. Future veterinary professionals might be trained to navigate vast digital platforms, interpreting data and integrating AI insights into their daily practice seamlessly. This evolution in training signifies an exciting time for education in veterinary sciences.

In the realm of pet care, the next decade is set to see a rise in smart home technologies tailored for animals. Imagine homes where AI-driven systems keep pets safe, monitor their health in real-time, and cater to their dietary and exercise needs with precision. Such innovations will not only enhance the well-being of domestic animals but will also improve the relationship between pets and their humans.

However, the road to AI ubiquity in veterinary medicine will not be without its challenges. Resistance to new technologies due to fears of the unknown, job displacement, or economic barriers will need addressing. Overcoming such obstacles will require strategic integration plans that involve stakeholders at all levels, ensuring that the benefits of AI are realized across the board.

In summary, as we look to the horizon, the future of AI in animal healthcare holds remarkable promise. Propelled by continuous advancements and the increasing synergy between technological and veterinary expertise, the next decade is set to manifest a healthcare revolution. By transforming how diagnoses are made, treatments are devised, and care is delivered, AI will play a central role in writing the next chapter in animal health, creating a world where animals thrive like never before.

Chapter 22:
AI and Public Perception in Veterinary Care

In recent years, the intersection of artificial intelligence and veterinary care has intrigued not just industry professionals, but the public at large. As AI increasingly plays a pivotal role in transforming animal healthcare, understanding and gauging public perception becomes critical. Many embrace these advancements with optimism, marveling at AI's potential to enhance diagnostics and tailor treatments. Yet, there are apprehensions—ranging from the accuracy of AI systems to concerns about data privacy. It's not uncommon for pet owners to find themselves weighing the benefits of cutting-edge AI solutions against their inherent uncertainties. Therefore, ongoing education is essential to demystify AI's applications and assuage fears. By fostering an open dialogue and promoting transparent practices, veterinarians and tech developers can work collaboratively to ensure that AI is not only a tool for advancement but also a trusted ally in the wider community. This dynamic landscape offers opportunities to build trust through empathy and understanding, ensuring AI-driven care becomes seamlessly integrated into our expectations for the future of veterinary medicine.

Educating the Public

In our rapidly evolving world, the role of artificial intelligence in veterinary medicine is burgeoning with promise. Yet, as with any transformative technology, the key to its successful integration lies not only in its adoption by professionals but also in its understanding by the general public. Educating people about AI's role in veterinary care is crucial for building trust and fostering acceptance. This chapter is dedicated to exploring ways to inform and engage the public about AI's contributions to animal health and well-being.

First and foremost, clear and accessible communication is vital. Often, the barrier to understanding lies in the complex jargon and technical specifics that accompany AI discussions. To combat this, we must endeavor to convey AI concepts in relatable terms. For instance, comparing AI algorithms to something as familiar as a recipe—where each set of instructions builds towards a final dish—can demystify how AI processes information. This form of metaphorical explanation can transform esoteric topics into digestible narratives that resonate with broader audiences.

Moreover, leveraging multimedia platforms can greatly aid in education initiatives. From informational videos to interactive webinars, utilizing these tools can help engage different learning preferences, ensuring a wider grasp among the audience. Imagine a series of short videos where veterinarians and AI experts jointly discuss the improvements in veterinary diagnostics. These videos could highlight real-life success stories, illustrating the tangible benefits of AI in practice, such as faster diagnostics and personalized treatment plans for beloved pets.

Community outreach programs can play a pivotal role in transforming public perception. Hosting events where technology meets touch—such as open house days at clinics or interactive exhibits at pet fairs—can create firsthand experiences of AI's capabilities. These events might showcase AI-assisted imaging tools used in diagnostics or wearable technology for pet health monitoring, allowing individuals to see and understand AI's benefits in a tangible and immediate way.

Another innovative approach is developing partnerships with educational institutions. By integrating AI education into veterinary and animal sciences curricula, future generations of pet owners and animal lovers can emerge with a foundational understanding of AI's competencies and limitations. This not only bolsters public knowledge but also encourages a culture of informed advocacy, where individuals can make knowledgeable decisions about their animal's healthcare options.

Addressing public concerns and misconceptions is an integral part of this educational mission. Misunderstandings about AI often stem from fears—rooted in science fiction narratives or misinformation—of losing the human element in veterinary care, or the ethical considerations surrounding AI use. It is essential to openly discuss these issues, perhaps through forums or online platforms where experts can address fears directly, providing facts that differentiate between Hollywood scenarios and reality.

Additionally, fostering a narrative that emphasizes AI as a supplementary, rather than a replacement, tool in veterinary medicine can alleviate fears. By framing AI technologies as allies in enhancing the ability of veterinarians to detect diseases earlier and customize treatment plans for individual animals, we reinforce the narrative that AI complements—aids and augments—human expertise rather than replaces it.

Storytelling can also be a powerful vehicle for educating the public. Case studies highlighting successful AI interventions in animal healthcare can act as inspirational tales that underline AI's potential. Whether it's a story of a wild animal population being monitored more effectively through AI analytics or a life saved through an early diagnosis made possible by machine learning, narratives have the power to connect emotionally with audiences, thereby dismantling barriers of skepticism and fostering a culture of curiosity and acceptance.

Incorporating AI learning modules into public library systems and community centers could broaden access to AI education across varying socioeconomic landscapes. Offering free courses or informational packets can democratize knowledge, ensuring that understanding and acceptance of AI in veterinary care is not only relegated to those with advanced technological literacy or access to specific digital resources.

Ultimately, education is not a one-off effort but a continuous journey. As AI technology evolves, so should our efforts to educate the public about its changing landscape. This involves maintaining regular updates through newsletters, online blogs, or podcasts, keeping the conversation ongoing and relevant. An informed public is an empowered one, capable of making decisions that align with both progressive veterinary practices and the welfare of their four-legged family members.

In conclusion, educating the public about AI in veterinary care promises to enhance both the field's development and the health of countless animals. Through creative communication, community engagement, and a commitment to transparency, we can nurture a collective understanding that opens doors to the incredible possibilities AI offers, ensuring a future where humans and technology harmoniously improve the lives of our animal companions.

Addressing Concerns and Misunderstandings

As we forge ahead into a future where artificial intelligence plays an ever-growing role in veterinary medicine, it's crucial to address common concerns and misunderstandings that can arise. Misinformation and hesitation are to be expected with any burgeoning technology, and AI is no exception. To fully harness its potential, it's important that we demystify AI for the skeptics, offering clarity, assurance, and a roadmap to its ethical and beneficial use.

A predominant concern is that AI could replace veterinarians, leading to job loss and a reduction in human-to-animal interaction. This fear, though understandable, doesn't account for AI's design as a supportive tool rather than a replacement. AI is intended to complement the skills of veterinarians, not substitute them. It's leveraging AI's strengths, such as data processing and pattern recognition, to improve accuracy and efficiency in diagnostics and treatment options. The human element remains irreplaceable, especially in offering empathy, intuition, and decision-making in unpredictable situations.

Another layer of misunderstanding revolves around AI's accuracy and reliability. While AI systems can process vast amounts of data with remarkable speed and precision, they are only as good as the data fed into them. There's concern about biases in AI algorithms, potentially leading to skewed results if not carefully managed. Ensuring that AI is trained on diverse and comprehensive datasets can mitigate these risks, increasing trust and reliability in its outputs. Vigilant human oversight also plays a vital role in maintaining AI's integrity, as professionals can intervene if anomalies arise.

Data privacy and security also crop up frequently in conversations about AI. Pet owners naturally worry about their animals' health data being handled ethically and securely. Veterinarians and AI developers need to work hand in hand to implement stringent data protection measures. By establishing transparent policies about data use and obtaining informed consent, they can help alleviate privacy concerns. Moreover, secure data storage and robust encryption methods should be standard protocol, ensuring sensitive information is safeguarded at all times.

There's a conceptual barrier when it comes to comprehending how AI functions. For some, AI seems like an abstract, almost magical entity, which can lead to skepticism or fear about its role. Veterinary professionals serving as educators can bridge this gap by explaining AI in relatable terms, emphasizing its logic-driven processes. By demystifying AI, they can build trust, illustrating how it increases the accuracy of diagnoses and enhances treatment plans, thus improving overall outcomes for animals.

The availability and cost of AI technologies also worry veterinarians and pet owners alike. Small practices may feel particularly burdened by the potential costs associated with integrating advanced AI systems. However, it's crucial to highlight that, in the long term, AI can lead to cost savings through improved efficiency, accurate diagnostics, and reduced trial-and-error in treatment plans. There are also scalable AI solutions that offer entry-level options for practices of various sizes, potentially providing a stepping stone toward more comprehensive adoption.

Given that AI development is ongoing, concerns over the longevity and consistent support for AI systems are valid. Veterinarians rely on the assurance that tech advancements maintain their relevance and receive regular updates to address emerging needs or issues. Establishing partnerships with leading AI firms can offer real-time support and consistent system enhancements, thus solidifying AI's position as a reliable fixture in veterinary care.

In addressing concerns about AI's role in emergency veterinary care, it's important to emphasize its capability to process information swiftly and support rapid decision-making. However, it should be clear that AI doesn't navigate these crises alone; instead, it acts in concert with human expertise. Veterinarians provide the necessary judgment and empathy in emergency circumstances, ensuring that AI remains a tool that enhances, rather than eclipses, human intervention.

Misunderstandings can also stem from cultural or generational differences in adopting new technologies. Older generations may be hesitant compared to younger cohorts who grew up in a digital world. Offering comprehensive training sessions and fostering environments where questions are encouraged can facilitate smoother transitions into AI-integrated practices. Sharing success stories and tangible benefits serves as a motivational tool, demonstrating AI's practical advantages in everyday veterinary settings.

In summary, addressing concerns and misunderstandings about AI in veterinary care involves open communication, ongoing education, and active collaboration. By dispelling myths and offering reassurance through transparency and demonstrable success, veterinary professionals can earn public trust. This transformative journey in animal healthcare boils down to blending AI's technological prowess with the compassion and care that defines veterinary medicine. Together, they form a promising alliance poised to enhance the health and well-being of animals, while elevating the capabilities of those who serve them.

Chapter 23:
Collaboration between AI Experts and Veterinarians

As technology continues to weave itself into the fabric of veterinary medicine, the collaboration between AI experts and veterinarians becomes a linchpin for innovation. This partnership brings together the analytical prowess of AI with the intuitive compassion of veterinary practitioners, creating a synergy that enhances animal healthcare. Teams blending AI specialists with seasoned veterinarians unlock new dimensions in diagnostics, treatment, and animal wellness. By addressing each other's knowledge gaps, these collaborations foster mutual growth and understanding. Together, they develop tools and protocols that are not only cutting-edge but also deeply empathetic, ensuring AI solutions are finely attuned to both medical needs and ethical considerations. This cooperative spirit is paving the way for advanced animal care, transforming the potential for what's possible in the clinics and beyond.

Building Effective Teams

In the rapidly evolving field of veterinary medicine enhanced by artificial intelligence, the importance of building effective teams cannot be overstated. Effective collaboration between AI experts and veterinarians is pivotal for harnessing the transformative power of AI technologies. These two groups bring distinct yet complementary skills to the table, forging partnerships that drive innovation and reshape animal healthcare.

AI experts possess technical knowledge and an understanding of the intricate algorithms and data science that underpin AI solutions. Meanwhile, veterinarians offer deep clinical insights and experience with animal health. By combining these expertise, multidisciplinary teams can create AI solutions that are both technically sound and practically applicable. Such collaboration involves continuous dialogue and exchange of ideas, allowing each profession to enhance its understanding of the other's domain.

Communication is the cornerstone of building effective teams. AI experts and veterinarians must develop a shared language to effectively discuss complex topics. This involves not just learning about each other's fields but also respecting and valuing different perspectives. When AI experts explain machine learning models, it should be in a manner that is accessible for non-specialists, including veterinarians. Similarly, veterinarians should present clinical challenges in a way that highlights specific areas where AI can make a difference.

Creating an environment that fosters curiosity and openness is key. Team members should feel encouraged to ask questions, challenge assumptions, and propose novel approaches without fear of judgment. In such a setting, team members can freely brainstorm and explore innovative ideas that might otherwise go unnoticed. When creativity is encouraged, new solutions to longstanding problems in animal health can emerge, leading to breakthroughs in diagnostics, treatment, and animal care.

One effective strategy for building successful teams is to establish clear goals and roles from the outset. When each team member understands their contributions and how these contributions fit into the larger picture, workflow is smoother and productivity increases.

Clear objectives help align efforts and focus on what truly matters for the success of AI-driven veterinary projects.

Moreover, a balance between autonomy and collaboration is crucial. Each professional should have the freedom to contribute ideas independently while remaining engaged in team activities. This balance allows for personal growth and fosters a spirit of innovation, while also ensuring that team efforts are cohesive and aligned with overall objectives.

Workshops and cross-disciplinary training sessions can also enhance team dynamics. By dedicating time to learn from each other, team members can bridge gaps in knowledge and build a more integrated understanding of AI applications in veterinary medicine. Such educational initiatives empower team members to become more adaptable and thoughtful in their approach to problem-solving.

Furthermore, the organizational culture surrounding these teams plays a significant role. Leadership needs to support and champion collaborative efforts. Providing resources, recognition, and incentives for innovative collaboration can motivate teams to push boundaries and strive for excellence. A supportive environment cultivates trust and accountability, which are essential components of any successful team.

Technology can serve as both a catalyst and a barrier to effective team building. It's crucial to choose tools that facilitate communication and project management, while also being mindful of potential challenges such as data privacy and security. Using tools tailored for collaborative work, such as shared digital workspaces and communication platforms, ensures seamless interaction and productivity.

Feedback loops are another essential aspect. Regularly reviewing team performance, reflecting on successes and areas for improvement, and making necessary adjustments, help maintain momentum and ensure continuous advancement toward common goals. Feedback should be constructive, focusing on solutions rather than problems, and it should be given and received in a spirit of mutual respect and encouragement.

Finally, celebrating achievements along the way strengthens team bonds and boosts morale. Recognizing and appreciating each member's contributions fosters a sense of community, which is vital for long-term collaboration. Celebrations can take many forms, from informal gatherings to formal recognition ceremonies, and they serve as reminders of the collective success achieved through united efforts.

Building effective teams in the intersection of AI and veterinary medicine isn't just about combining expertise; it's about creating a culture that values diversity, fosters innovation, and works towards shared goals. When AI experts and veterinarians successfully collaborate, they pioneer new frontiers in animal healthcare, ultimately benefiting animals and their caregivers alike.

Bridging the Knowledge Gap

In the fast-evolving landscape of artificial intelligence (AI) within veterinary medicine, one challenge that looms large is the knowledge gap between AI experts and veterinarians. For AI to truly enhance animal healthcare, these two distinct groups must find a common language and understanding. This section delves into the necessity and strategies for bridging this gap, a crucial step toward reaping the full benefits of AI in veterinary contexts.

Veterinarians, with their deep understanding of animal physiology and clinical expertise, are indispensable in the development of effective AI applications in animal health. They bring a practical perspective that is essential for creating tools that are not just technologically advanced but also clinically relevant. On the other hand, AI experts possess the technical know-how to design systems capable of handling complex data analysis, pattern recognition, and predictive modeling. The challenge lies in merging these disparate knowledge bases into a cohesive working relationship where both sides appreciate and utilize each other's expertise.

One of the fundamental barriers in collaboration is language. Veterinarians and AI specialists often speak in jargon specific to their fields. While veterinarians use terms deeply rooted in biology and medicine, AI experts may default to a lexicon filled with technical algorithms and computational processes. To overcome this communication barrier, interdisciplinary education and workshops can serve as a platform where both parties can learn the basics of each other's field. Such initiatives ensure that veterinarians gain a better grasp of what AI tools can do, while AI experts learn about the practical issues veterinarians face in their day-to-day practice.

Moreover, fostering a culture of continual learning and adaptability within veterinary practices is paramount. Veterinary professionals can benefit from training sessions and resources that not only teach them about AI technologies but also how to interpret and question AI-derived data critically. They shouldn't be passive recipients of technology, but active participants in the co-development of AI solutions. This involvement not only enhances their trust in these systems but also ensures that the AI tools developed are tailored to address real veterinary challenges.

In the same vein, AI developers must seek to understand the ethical and practical considerations that veterinarians muster daily. Building AI tools that respect animal welfare, adhere to ethical norms, and integrate seamlessly into existing veterinary workflows is essential. When AI developers appreciate these considerations, the tools they create are not disruptive but instead act as valuable extensions of the veterinarians' capabilities.

Joint projects between universities, technology companies, and veterinary schools can act as incubators for collaborative innovation. Such projects might focus on developing specific AI applications in diagnostics or treatment protocols, with a structured framework for feedback and iteration. This collaborative model not only fuels innovation but also builds partnerships and camaraderie between AI experts and veterinarians. When professionals from these diverse fields collaborate closely, they cultivate a shared vision that prioritizes animal welfare and delivers tangible benefits to animal health.

To further facilitate collaboration, it is beneficial to establish interdisciplinary teams within veterinary practices and research institutions. These teams can include veterinarians, AI specialists, data scientists, and even ethicists to ensure a balanced approach to AI implementation. By working together, they can address various facets of AI application—from technical feasibility and clinical effectiveness to ethical implications and user adoption.

Transparency in AI development is another crucial element in bridging the knowledge gap. AI systems must be understood, tested, and validated collaboratively. Veterinarians should be involved in every phase, from ideation to implementation. Engaging them in the validation and testing phases ensures that AI tools not only function as intended but also meet the clinical needs encountered in everyday veterinary practice. Allowing access to data, methodologies, and outcomes ensures that veterinarians can trust the systems, leading to increased acceptance and reliance on AI technologies.

From the perspective of continuous professional development, hosting seminars, conferences, and symposiums that bring together AI experts and veterinarians can foster dialogue and knowledge exchange. These events should encourage open discussion of successes and failures, with an emphasis on collaborative learning. Success stories can motivate further integration, while lessons from failure can provide critical insights into potential pitfalls and areas for improvement.

Additionally, educational institutions must adapt to these changes by offering programs that blend veterinary science and AI literacy. By incorporating elements of data science, machine learning, and AI ethics into veterinary education, a new generation of veterinarians will be better equipped to work alongside AI experts. Simultaneously, AI curricula should include modules that familiarize technologists with the fundamentals of veterinary medicine.

Looking toward the future, it is exciting to envision a realm where AI and veterinary medicine coalesce into a seamless ecosystem characterized by mutual respect, shared goals, and collaborative innovation. The bridging of this knowledge gap presents both a challenge and an opportunity for visionary change that can redefine the boundaries of what's possible in animal healthcare.

Chapter 24:
AI for Pets in the Home

Integrating artificial intelligence into our homes is not just for human convenience anymore; it's also transforming how we care for our beloved pets. AI-driven devices like smart feeders, voice-activated treat dispensers, and intelligent litter boxes are weaving seamlessly into the smart home ecosystem, making it easier for pet owners to monitor and enhance their furry friends' well-being. Imagine a world where your pet's mood, dietary needs, and health conditions can be continuously tracked and optimized using AI algorithms. This is no longer a futuristic dream but a growing reality that empowers pet parents to offer more personalized care and timely interventions. With these technological marvels, pets can enjoy an enriched environment that adapts to their unique needs, helping to reduce stress and improve quality of life. As these systems evolve, so does the potential for a deeper understanding of our pets' lives, offering new ways to fortify the bond between humans and animals. Embracing AI in the home means stepping into a world where pet care becomes more intuitive and dynamic, ensuring our furry companions live healthier, happier lives.

Integrating Smart Home Technologies

The integration of smart home technologies into pet care isn't just a fanciful notion—it's rapidly becoming a practical reality that offers manifold benefits for enhancing pet well-being. These advancements aren't about replacing the personal touch that pet owners cherish, but amplifying their abilities to deliver care that's both more efficient and personalized. AI-enabled devices, such as automated feeders and smart cameras, have begun to transform the way pets are monitored and cared for in domestic settings.

The core advantage of smart home technologies is their capacity for real-time monitoring. Imagine a pet camera equipped with AI that not only captures video but can also analyze your pet's movements and alert you to unusual patterns. This is where the true magic happens. If your dog is pacing more than usual, it could send you an alert, suggesting the need for a wellness check. Such proactive alerts—rooted in predictive analytics—can be revolutionary in detecting issues before they become serious.

Incorporating intelligent feeding systems is another exciting development. These systems don't just dispense food automatically but can adjust feeding schedules based on your pet's age, weight, and health conditions. AI-driven feeders can even suggest dietary adjustments by analyzing your pet's eating habits over time. Imagine a system that balances nutritional needs in real-time, helping manage everything from weight to dietary deficiencies. It's not hard to see how such technologies can vastly improve your pet's overall health.

Additionally, smart home technology is invaluable for managing and regulating environmental factors that impact a pet's comfort and health. AI-integrated thermostats and lighting systems can adjust environmental conditions based on your pet's breed and specific needs. Certain breeds are more sensitive to temperature fluctuations, and having an automated system ensure optimal conditions can prevent unnecessary stress and health complications.

The flexibility and scalability of these technologies also mean they can be tailored to meet the specific requirements of various types of pets. Whether you have a cat, dog, or more exotic animal, these systems can adjust to provide the most appropriate care. Moreover, AI technology can learn and evolve with your pet, adapting to their changing needs and preferences over time. It's akin to having a customizable care plan that grows with your pet.

Voice recognition is another thrilling facet of this tech revolution. Voice-activated toys and training aids can respond to commands not just from owners but can also be programmed to react to your pet's vocalizations. Imagine a device that can understand when your cat meows for attention and responds by activating a toy or playing soothing music. This personalized interaction can enrich your pet's life, providing mental stimulation and emotional comfort.

However, as with any technological advancement, integrating AI-powered smart home technologies comes with challenges—primarily around privacy and security. Devices designed to monitor pets, like cameras, need robust cybersecurity measures to prevent unauthorized access. Furthermore, while these technologies offer significant advantages, they should always complement, not replace, hands-on pet care and vet consultations. Owners must still be actively involved in their pets' lives, using these tools to enhance their caregiving, not as a substitute for personal interaction and professional guidance.

Smart home technologies also offer an intriguing opportunity for veterinarians and pet owners to collaborate more closely. Devices can transmit data not just to the owner, but directly to the veterinarian, allowing for a more integrated approach to monitoring pet health. This collaboration can lead to quicker diagnoses and more efficient treatments. Sharing insights with a vet from your home becomes seamless, offering unprecedented continuity in animal healthcare.

These advancements also hold potential for a more connected community of pet owners and professionals. By sharing data and experiences, pet owners can contribute to a larger body of knowledge concerning animal health and behavior. This collective intelligence can drive further innovations, encouraging manufacturers to build even more refined and effective AI tools for pet care.

The expansion of AI and smart technologies into the realm of pet care isn't just a tech-driven trend but represents a paradigm shift towards more holistic and integrative animal care. By embracing these technologies, pet owners can ensure not just the physical health of their companions, but also their psychological well-being, making their lives richer and more fulfilling. As these technologies continue to evolve, the possibilities seem as limitless and enriching as the unconditional love we share with our pets.

Enhancing Pet Well-Being

The integration of artificial intelligence into home environments is not just redefining human experiences; it's also crafting new pathways for enhancing the well-being of our furry companions. Imagine a world where AI-driven technologies enable pets to live healthier, more enriched lives. In this evolving landscape, AI is stepping up as a vital ally in understanding and catering to the nuanced needs of our pets, transforming everyday caregiving into a much more personalized experience.

AI technologies are revolutionizing how we monitor pet health and behavior in the home setting. With the help of smart collars and home devices, pet owners gain insights into their pet's activity levels, sleep patterns, and even mood fluctuations. These AI-infused gadgets interpret real-time data, allowing us to identify potential health issues before they become significant problems. If a cat's activity level drops suddenly or a dog's sleep becomes erratic, an alert can prompt further attention, avoiding unnecessary distress for the animal. By translating data into actionable insights, these technologies ensure pets receive the care they need in a timely manner.

Moreover, AI-driven apps are rapidly advancing to evaluate and enhance pet mental stimulation. These applications can recommend interactive games and activities based on an animal's breed, age, and personality. Such tailored recommendations ensure that pets remain engaged and mentally stimulated, which is crucial for their overall health. Playtime is more than just fun for pets; it's an essential element of their well-being, helping to stave off boredom and reduce anxiety-induced behaviors.

The fusion of AI and nutrition is another exciting frontier. With AI's analytical power, dietary plans can be formulated to align closely with veterinary recommendations and the specific health needs of each pet. Automated insights from AI can suggest dietary adjustments if a dog gains weight too quickly or if a cat's energy levels don't align with its nutritional intake. This proactive approach to diet planning helps in maintaining an optimal weight and meeting the unique nutritional needs of each pet, supporting longevity and vitality.

Beyond physical health, AI technologies are also set to revolutionize how we tackle behavioral issues. Analyzing patterns in behavior helps identify stressors or environmental factors contributing to issues like aggression or excessive barking. By understanding triggers through AI analyses, we can tailor interventions that might include training programs or changes in the pet's environment. With AI's assistance, these solutions become more predictable and effective, delivering results that are both humane and science-backed.

Importantly, AI is not working alone; it gathers and processes data that can be seamlessly shared with veterinarians. This collaboration enriches the veterinary consultation process by providing precise, data-driven insights into a pet's home life. Such information is invaluable in diagnosing conditions and tailoring treatment plans. Therefore, AI forms a bridge, enabling closer cooperation between pet owners and veterinary professionals.

Within homes, AI can create safe environments that adapt to pets' needs. Smart homes integrated with AI can monitor temperature, humidity, and light, ensuring optimal living conditions for pets. For example, houses can automatically adjust settings to provide comfort for dogs on hot days or ensure proper lighting for birds in the evening. It's about creating living spaces that cater to pets, making homes not just places they live in, but environments that actively support their well-being.

Despite the technological prowess, the key lies in designing systems that are user-friendly and intuitive. For technology to be effective, it needs to be accessible and understandable for end users, which in this case is the pet owner. Usability ensures that pet owners can seamlessly integrate technology into their daily routines without feeling overwhelmed.

Furthermore, the trust in AI and its applications is reinforced through transparency and consistent results. As owners witness firsthand the improvements in their pets' well-being, from increased energy levels to a clearer understanding of their needs, the reliance on and acceptance of AI in everyday pet care naturally grows.

In this journey towards enriching pet lives through technology, ethical considerations must not be sidelined. It's essential to ensure that all AI interventions respect animal welfare and align with the highest ethical standards. The goal is to use technology as a tool to enhance life, not control it. Thus, developers and users alike must continually assess and recalibrate their approaches to maintain a balance between innovation and care.

Ultimately, enhancing pet well-being through AI is about empowering pet owners with tools that provide deeper insights and more precise care options. It's about reshaping pet care into a dynamic and responsive practice that evolves with the needs of each individual animal. As AI technology progresses, the opportunities to transform and elevate pet well-being will only expand, opening new realms of possibility for fostering healthier, happier lives for our beloved animals.

Chapter 25:
Overcoming Challenges in AI Adoption

Adopting artificial intelligence in veterinary medicine is transformative, yet it comes with its own set of hurdles that practitioners must navigate to harness its full potential. AI's promise of enhanced diagnostic precision and customized care meets real-world obstacles like technological resistance, cost concerns, and the complexity of integrating AI systems into traditional workflows. Veterinarians, often entrenched in conventional practices, may initially feel overwhelmed by the prospects and challenges presented by AI. Bridging this gap requires a concerted effort in education and change management, ensuring that everyone involved understands both the benefits and limitations of AI applications in animal healthcare. Success hinges on fostering an open culture where continuous learning is encouraged, and interdisciplinary collaboration is the norm. By addressing initial hesitations with clear communication and support, the veterinary field can confidently transition into an AI-augmented future, ultimately revolutionizing animal care by making it more efficient, personalized, and far-reaching.

Addressing Resistance and Misconceptions

As artificial intelligence continues to revolutionize veterinary medicine, resistance and misconceptions can hinder its adoption. These barriers are often rooted in fear, misinformation, and a lack of understanding of AI's capabilities and limitations. To effectively integrate AI into animal healthcare, it's critical to address these resistances head-on and demystify the technology.

One significant misconception about AI in veterinary practices is that it will replace veterinarians and their staff. This concern is understandable but largely unfounded. AI is designed to augment the capabilities of veterinary professionals, not to replace them. It can handle time-consuming tasks like data analysis and pattern recognition, allowing vets to focus on the nuanced aspects of care that require human empathy and decision-making. For example, while AI can help diagnose diseases through imaging analysis, it lacks the ability to console anxious pet owners or make ethical decisions in treatment plans.

The fear of losing the human touch is another common resistance point. Veterinary care is inherently compassionate, and the idea that machines could take over this role is unsettling for many. However, AI can enhance human-animal interactions rather than diminish them. With AI handling complex data, veterinarians have more time to engage with their patients, understand their needs, and provide personalized care. In truth, AI can act as an enabler, bringing veterinary teams closer to animals and their owners by freeing up time and resources.

Data privacy and security concerns also play a significant role in resistance to AI adoption. The veterinary community, much like its human healthcare counterpart, handles sensitive data, and the idea of feeding this data into AI systems can seem risky. However, advancements in machine learning have included stringent measures for data protection. Encryption, secure access protocols, and strict compliance with data protection regulations are integral parts of AI systems. Educating stakeholders on these security measures could alleviate many concerns.

Some veterinarians worry that AI is just a passing fad or that it's being implemented prematurely, without sufficient evidence of its efficacy. This skepticism often stems from a misunderstanding of how AI technologies develop. Machine learning, a core component of AI, relies on large datasets to improve over time. As more veterinary data becomes available, AI's diagnostic accuracy and therapeutic recommendations will enhance, further validating its place in routine practices. Highlighting successful case studies and ongoing research can bolster confidence and demonstrate AI's tangible benefits.

Another common misconception is that AI is a one-size-fits-all solution. In reality, AI applications in veterinary medicine need to be carefully tailored to specific needs and contexts. Successfully integrating AI requires a collaborative approach where veterinary professionals work with technologists to customize AI tools that address the unique challenges of different species and medical conditions. Recognizing AI's role as a versatile tool, rather than a panacea, can help recalibrate expectations and build a more nuanced understanding of its potential.

Despite these challenges, there's a growing body of evidence supporting AI's positive impact on veterinary practices. Its ability to analyze vast amounts of data quickly leads to quicker, more accurate diagnoses and treatment plans. Moreover, AI can continuously learn and adapt, improving its performance as it gains access to more real-world data. By actively engaging with the veterinary profession's particular needs, AI offers innovative solutions that drive advancement rather than detracting from traditional practices.

Addressing resistance to AI also involves engaging in continuous education and transparent communication. Providing training and resources to veterinary professionals can help them understand and utilize AI more effectively. Workshops, seminars, and online courses offer opportunities for veterinarians to learn about AI's tools, capabilities, and limitations. Likewise, transparent discussions about AI's role, benefits, and potential pitfalls can help clear the air of myths and foster a culture of trust and collaboration.

Ultimately, addressing resistance involves advocating for an AI co-existence strategy rather than an AI replacement strategy. This means acknowledging that while AI can handle some tasks better, it cannot replicate the intuition, creativity, and empathy of humans. By creating environments where technology and human expertise harmoniously coexist, the veterinary field can take full advantage of AI's capabilities to improve animal health outcomes.

As the line between tech and touch continues to blur, demystifying AI can help vet professionals and animal lovers alike embrace its potential. By doing so, the journey toward its full adoption becomes one of collaboration, innovation, and meaningful improvement in animal healthcare.

Strategies for Successful Integration

As we delve into the realm of artificial intelligence (AI) in veterinary medicine, success hinges not just on innovation but on adept integration. The road to effective AI adoption is paved with strategic planning and clear understanding. Those in the veterinary field who are open to leveraging AI have a unique opportunity to transform their practices. Yet, it requires deliberate actions and thoughtful approaches to ensure this technology aligns with the goals of veterinary care.

First and foremost, a clear understanding of the potential benefits and limitations of AI is essential. Veterinary professionals must familiarize themselves with how AI technologies like machine learning and predictive analytics can specifically enhance diagnostics, treatment, and animal care. Defining specific roles that AI can play in their practice can help veterinarians tailor their integration strategies. This involves identifying bottlenecks or challenges within their current systems that AI could address effectively, such as improving diagnostic accuracy or optimizing treatment timelines.

The next step is to conduct thorough training for all staff members who will interact with AI systems. Just as important as the technology itself is the ability of staff to use AI tools effectively. Training programs should encompass not only technical skills but also foster an understanding of AI's role in enhancing clinical outcomes. By building confidence and competence around AI technologies, veterinary teams can minimize resistance and harness AI's capabilities to their full potential.

Moreover, integrating AI requires a careful calibration of workflows. Traditional practices may need to be adapted in order to incorporate AI efficiently without causing disruptions. Identifying essential processes that can be automated and ensuring seamless information flow between AI systems and human operators is vital. This reduces the risk of bottlenecks and enhances the overall efficiency of the veterinary practice. For example, AI-powered diagnostic tools must integrate smoothly with existing medical record systems to provide comprehensive insights and ensure practitioners can access the most accurate and up-to-date information.

Partnerships and collaborations with AI experts and technology providers can play a crucial role in overcoming integration challenges. Such collaborations facilitate knowledge exchange and offer support during and after implementation. Engaging with technology partners who understand the nuances of veterinary medicine can lead to customized solutions that align more closely with the specific needs and workflows of a veterinary clinic.

Regular evaluation and feedback mechanisms should be established to continually assess the effectiveness of the AI systems in use. The rapidly evolving nature of AI technologies means that constant review and adaptation are necessary. Veterinary practices should expect to iterate on their use of technology, making iterative adjustments based on practical experience and feedback from both staff and clients. Continuous improvement ensures that AI remains an asset rather than a liability, enhancing rather than impeding veterinary care.

Transparency with clients about the role of AI in their pets' care is another critical consideration. Educating pet owners on how AI tools contribute to diagnosis or treatment allows for informed decisions and fosters trust. When clients understand the benefits AI brings to the table, they are more likely to embrace the technology's role in the well-being of their animals. Clear communication about how AI is used, and its potential impacts can alleviate fears and enhance satisfaction with care services.

Investing in the right technologies is another essential facet of successful AI integration. Whether choosing AI for remote monitoring, diagnostics, or nutritional planning, investment decisions should be informed by a balanced assessment of cost versus potential value. In this endeavor, a thorough cost-benefit analysis is indispensable. Practices need to consider not only the initial expenditure but the potential long-term savings and improved clinical outcomes AI can deliver.

Finally, the broader ethical implications of AI in veterinary medicine must be continually considered. Responsible use of AI involves respecting the autonomy of veterinary professionals while ensuring animal welfare remains the focus. Adhering to established ethical standards when implementing AI ensures that technological advances do not come at the cost of care quality. Incorporating an ethical framework into the integration process can help navigate potential challenges and reinforce AI's position as a force for good in animal healthcare.

Conclusion

In the ever-evolving landscape of veterinary medicine, artificial intelligence stands as a beacon of transformative potential. The integration of AI into animal healthcare is not just a technological leap; it's a profound change in how we approach the diagnosis, treatment, and overall well-being of our animal companions. As we've explored throughout this book, AI is reshaping the veterinary field in countless ways, enhancing the lives of both animals and the professionals who care for them.

The journey through AI in veterinary medicine is one of discovery and innovation. We've seen how AI-driven diagnostics can lead to earlier detection of diseases, allowing for timely interventions and better prognoses. Automated imaging and advanced analysis are enabling veterinarians to see beyond traditional diagnostic boundaries, offering insights that were once the realm of speculation.

Tailored treatment plans, facilitated by AI, present a new era in personalized medicine for animals. No longer are treatments solely based on generalized protocols; AI algorithms analyze individual histories and genetic data, crafting therapies that cater to the specific needs of each patient. This shift from centralized therapy to individualized care signifies a major advance in how veterinary medicine is practiced.

In surgical suites, AI is becoming an indispensable partner. It's not just about precision; it's about redefining what's possible. With the aid of robotics and AI-assisted technologies, complex procedures become not only feasible but safer. As outcomes improve, both animals and their caretakers benefit from reduced recovery times and enhanced postoperative success.

A significant frontier where AI is making its presence felt is in research and development. AI's capability to sift through vast amounts of data accelerates drug discovery and revolutionizes clinical trials. This isn't merely about speed; it's about refining accuracy and enhancing the relevance of results, making strides in veterinary pharmacology that will have lasting impacts.

Telemedicine, supported by AI, breaks down geographical and resource barriers. With remote diagnostics and virtual consultations, veterinary care is expanding its reach. This technological leap increases accessibility, bringing quality animal care to underserved areas and improving the standards of global animal health.

The conservation of wildlife and care for exotic species also benefit enormously from AI. Monitoring technologies powered by AI allow for real-time tracking of wildlife populations and contribute valuable data to conservation efforts. These innovations aren't just saving animals; they're preserving ecosystems and biodiversity for future generations.

The application of predictive analytics in veterinary practices signifies a proactive approach to animal health management. By forecasting health trends, practitioners can anticipate issues before they arise, allowing for preventive measures that support long-term animal health. This forecasting ability transforms the traditionally reactive nature of healthcare into a forward-thinking discipline.

AI's impact on nutrition and dietary planning for animals introduces a nuanced approach to health management that considers the dietary needs of individual animals, optimizing their health and performance. As dietary insights evolve, AI technologies monitor nutritional intake, ensuring well-rounded and balanced diets for all species under care.

We've also explored the revolutionary impact of smart technology in animal monitoring. Wearable devices provide real-time health tracking, allowing for instantaneous reactions to health changes. By constantly monitoring vital signs, activity levels, and other health metrics, these devices ensure that animals receive care informed by up-to-the-minute data.

Understanding animal behavior through AI tools not only offers novel insights into the social and psychological aspects of animals but also aids in addressing behavioral issues with unprecedented depth and precision. Our relationship with animals is deepened when we understand and respond to their behavioral cues effectively.

As with any technological advancement, the integration of AI in veterinary medicine carries significant ethical considerations. Balancing the promise of innovation with ethical responsibility is crucial. Maintaining a focus on caring while utilizing AI technologies aims to ensure ethical standards maintain parity with technological advancements.

There's no question that AI is also altering veterinary education, equipping the next generation of veterinarians with the tools they need to harness these digital possibilities fully. From AI-enhanced learning tools to the incorporation of cutting-edge practices, the educational landscape is transforming, preparing students for a future where AI is an integral part of animal healthcare.

In times of emergency and crisis, AI can be an ally in rapid triage and decision-making processes, enabling swifter responses that can often spell the difference between life and death. The application of AI drives forward-thinking responses, making emergency care more efficient and effective.

For large animals and livestock, AI optimizes farm management, boosting productivity and ensuring the health of herds and flocks. By monitoring livestock in real-time, AI solutions enhance health outcomes and contribute to sustainable farming practices, driving agricultural efficiency that benefits food supply chains globally.

As we look to the future, the convergence of AI and veterinary genomics holds promise for groundbreaking developments in genetic understanding and management. The potential for genetic improvements and preventive health strategies is vast, forecasted to reduce hereditary illnesses and improve overall animal health.

End-of-life care for animals is another area where AI is making significant strides, offering compassionate support solutions for both animals and their human counterparts. The delicate balance between technology and empathy nurtures dignity in final care, echoing the commitment to humane treatment at all stages of life.

Legal and regulatory landscapes surrounding AI continue to evolve, ensuring compliance and safety in its application within veterinary practices. These frameworks are paramount in safeguarding ethical standards and securing public trust in the technological advancements utilized in animal healthcare.

Financially, the integration of AI into veterinary practices opens new avenues for cost-effective care while attracting investment opportunities. By fostering a deeper understanding of AI's cost-benefit dynamics, practices can make informed decisions that enhance their operations and service offerings.

Awareness and education about AI's role in veterinary practices are crucial for overcoming public misconceptions and resistance to adoption. By fostering collaboration among AI experts and veterinarians, knowledge gaps are bridged, driving forward the effective implementation of AI technologies that benefit animals and their caregivers alike.

The future of AI in veterinary medicine is truly exciting. As developments accelerate, staying informed and adapting to these changes will be key to unlocking AI's full potential, ensuring that we continue to enhance the well-being of animals worldwide. The journey is ongoing, and the rewards promise to be as immense as the passions that drive those committed to this cause.

Appendix A:
Appendix

In this appendix, we'll touch on a number of vital resources, references, and supplementary materials that further illuminate the profound impact of artificial intelligence on veterinary medicine. This section is designed to be a springboard for further exploration, offering insights and pathways for those eager to delve deeper into the intricacies of AI's role in advancing animal health and care.

1. Key References and Further Reading

To fully appreciate the transformation AI is instigating in veterinary practices, it is beneficial to turn to various scholarly articles, industry reports, and books that detail these advancements. These references provide foundational knowledge and current findings:

Foundational Texts on AI and Machine Learning

Research Papers on AI Diagnostics in Veterinary Medicine

Case Studies of AI Implementation in Clinical Settings

Industry Reports on Emerging AI Technologies

Books Focusing on AI Ethics and Regulations

2. Tools and Technologies

The appendix outlines some of the technologies that are pivotal to the ongoing AI revolution in veterinary medicine:

Automated Diagnostic Tools

Advanced Imaging Technologies

Robotic Surgery Aids

Wearable Tracking Devices for Animals

AI-Driven Behavior Analysis Software

3. Organizations and Conferences

Engaging with professional organizations and attending specialized conferences can further enhance understanding and keep practitioners at the forefront of AI developments in veterinary care:

International Association for Veterinary AI

Global Veterinary AI Conference

Society for Veterinary Informatics

AI in Animal Health Symposiums

4. Developing Skills and Training

Continuing education and skill development are crucial for those in the veterinary field aiming to leverage AI effectively. Consider engaging with:

Online Courses on AI Applications in Healthcare

Workshops on Machine Learning for Veterinary Applications

Certification Programs in Veterinary Informatics

5. Ethical and Legal Considerations

Finally, the appendix reiterates the importance of understanding the ethical and legal frameworks surrounding AI use in veterinary settings. Staying informed about:

Ethical Guidelines for AI Use

Legal Standards and Compliance Requirements

Policy Statements from Veterinary Associations

This appendix serves as a gateway to a network of resources that can support and enrich the journey of veterinary professionals as AI continues to reshape the landscape of animal healthcare. It's an exciting era where technology and compassion converge to create new opportunities for enhancing the well-being of animals across the globe.